Lower Blood Pressure Without Drugs

By

Roger Mason

Lower Blood Pressure Without Drugs

by
Roger Mason

ISBN   1884820-82-4
9781884820823
Library of Congress Catalog Card #2008943289
Categories: 1. Health 2.Nutrition

Printed in the U.S.A.
1st Printing Spring 2009

Published by Safe Goods
561 Shunpike Road, Sheffield, MA 01257
(888) NATURE-1
(888)628-8731
www.safegoodspub.com

Contents

4

About This Book

This book is the most researched, comprehensive and effective book in print on lowering blood pressure in print. Here you find endless scientific, international, published clinical proof of everything you read. You don't lower blood pressure by covering up the symptoms with toxic, expensive drugs having serious side effects. These poisons shorten your life, and hurt the quality of your life. The vast majority of books on curing hypertension naturally simply do not work, and are full of misinformation.

Using natural medicine you treat the cause of your problems with diet and life style. *Diet and life style cure disease.* Diet and life style lower your blood pressure. Diet and life style are the only real cure. Diet, proven supplements, natural hormones, exercise, weekly fasting, refusing all prescription drugs and medical treatments, and cutting back or ending any bad habits (like coffee) is the only path to wellness. Read *Seven Steps to Natural Health* on page 84.

Americans, along with the Japanese, generally have the highest blood pressure levels of anyone. This is not merely due to stress. The key to understanding high blood pressure more than anything else is *insulin resistance.* Insulin resistance is the basic cause of high blood pressure. Here the body makes enough insulin, but the muscle cells no longer react well to it; they are resistant to the insulin. The main cause of this is our extreme consumption of various sugars. This is the real reason. Americans, on the average, hog down over 160 pounds of various sugars every year. We have no need for any sugar. No other country downs this much sugar. Never before in the history of the world has any society done this. No culture has ever consumed this many calories, this amount of simple sugars - or the many sugar substitutes. *Now one in three American children will grow up diabetic!* This is insane, yet accepted somehow. Now, one in three of our children will be diabetics.

Everything you need to know is in this factual, easy to read book. Be your own doctor and take responsibility for your health.

Overview

Essential hypertension is the most prevalent medical condition on the face of the earth. Over 65 million American adults have high blood pressure, defined as 140/90. Over 40 million more are "pre-hypertensive" defined as pressures over 120/80. Anti-hypertensive drugs are the third most common prescriptions written, only after cholesterol-lowering and pain relief. These toxic dangerous drugs merely cover up the symptoms, while leaving the causes ignored. One third of all American adults suffer from high blood pressure, and many of them go undiagnosed. This is not merely a Western phenomenon, but a worldwide one that affects poor rural people as well. Cardiovascular heart disease (CHD) is the biggest killer of all worldwide. Hypertension is the most prominent cardio-vascular condition of all. It does not need to be this way at all. This epidemic is completely unnecessary and easily avoided. High blood pressure is a major cause of stroke, heart attacks, congestive heart failure, kidney disease, and artery disease among other conditions.

Most people blame hypertension on stress. Stress is certainly a factor here, but not the main cause at all. It does not explain why some people cope with equal amounts of stress and don't raise their blood pressure. *Insulin resistance is the real cause more than any other factor.* More than anything, insulin resistance is caused by excessive intake of all simple sugars. Other major factors include obesity, lack of exercise, alcohol intake, excessive fat and protein intake, and undernutrition. We are overfed and undernourished. Now, even our children are suffering from hypertension, high cholesterol, and other heart and artery problems. This has never happened before. There is just no reason to have high blood pressure when you can make better food choices and get regular exercise. There is certainly no reason to resort to dangerous and expensive drugs when natural cures are so readily available.

This book is based on the last twenty years of international published research from *Chemical Abstracts.*

Chapter 1: About Hypertension

High blood pressure is the most epidemic disease on earth bar none. No medical condition approaches essential hypertension in numbers. In America alone there are over 100 million adults with pre-hypertension, or outright hypertension. This is classically defined as 140/90 readings, and pre-hypertension as 130/85. You have to go beyond these readings and know other parameters. Total cholesterol, triglycerides, uric acid, CRP, homocysteine, blood sugar, GTT, albumin, creatinine, SGOT, SGPT, and bilirubin are the twelve most important ones.

Age is the most important factor of all, because everyone gets old- if they're lucky. There is a direct correlation between age and incidence of hypertension. The older you get the higher your pressures generally. In developed countries however we are finding more and more problems with younger and younger people. Just as we are finding increasing problems with obesity, diabetes, high cholesterol, and other such problems usually associated with age, we are now finding hypertension even in children and adolescents.

Surprisingly, you will find high blood pressure levels even in third world countries, including rural areas where you would least expect it. A good example is the rural Nigerian people, who have little obesity, diabetes, or cholesterol problems, and smoking and coffee are not regular habits. Thirty percent of adults are hypertensive, even though, ironically, they have a very low incidence of CHD (cardiovascular disease). This is more proof we cannot reduce the problem down to stress, since there is usually little stress in rural people.

You'll find in this book that the main cause of hypertension is *insulin resistance*, where the body cells no longer respond well to normal amounts of insulin. This is basically caused by our outrageous intake of over 160 pounds of various simple sugars every year- more sugar than any other country eats.

Second to blood sugar dysmetabolism are various kidney

weaknesses and dysfunctions. These are basically caused by our intake of twice the protein we need, nearly all of which is animal, not plant, protein. Excessive added table salt adds to this problem, but is highly overrated as a cause. One-in-three American adults are now clinically obese, and obesity is a very powerful direct factor. Minerals are vital here, too, and we are very mineral deficient. Overfed and undernourished. The liver is also involved in blood pressure regulation. University Hospital in Switzerland said the problem starts as micro-albuminuria, then progresses to clinical proteinuria, to progressive chronic renal failure, to outright kidney disease.

The liver is our largest internal organ (technically our skin is our largest organ) and controls blood sugar by the release of glycogen into the blood. Liver problems are also strongly associated with blood pressure. SGPT, SGOT, and bilirubin levels are routinely checked during any comprehensive blood analysis. Liver problems are far too common in America due to three factors, 1) our 42 percent intake of saturated fats, 2) our overconsumption of alcohol, and 3) our inordinate intake of prescription and recreational drugs. City Hospital in England found hypertension clearly associated with elevated liver enzymes and fatty livers. The Affiliated Hospital in China found low bilirubin levels in hypertensive people.

Obesity is a pillar of hypertension, and most patients are over-weight. One-third of American adults are obese. *You must lose weight to lower blood pressure.* Americans eat twice the food they need. We literally eat for two people every day. Men only need about 1,800 calories, and women only about 1,200. That's all. Calorie restriction greatly improves blood pressures, not only through weight loss, but by less oxidative stress from overeating. The University of Colorado found low calorie diets (from low fat foods) lowered blood pressure in people with no other lifestyle changes.

Oxidative stress is also a major factor, where excessive free radicals cause damage to the entire body. We get almost no exercise anymore, and you must exercise to cure any kind of coronary or blood sugar condition. The answer to oxidative stress is better diet, fewer calories, regular exercise, and proven supplements especially antiox-

8

idants. Oxidative stress can be measured by MDA (malondialdehyde) or TBARS (thiobarbituric acid) blood levels, but this is not necessary at all. Seoul University in Korea found poor antioxidant status (TAS) and oxidative stress to be basic causes of high blood pressure, and correlated strongly with obesity. Doctors at the University of Montreal discovered the development of insulin resistance, the model of hypertension, was found to be prevented by chronic antioxidant therapies. Oxidative stress is a major pathogenic factor in hypertension.

Most all doctors recommend one of five classes of dangerous, toxic drugs that cover up a symptom, and make your health worse. This ever changing array of pharmaceutical poisons includes diuretics, beta blockers, ACE inhibitors, angiotensin II receptor antagonists, and calcium channel blockers. Tens of billions of dollars of these toxins are sold worldwide every year, especially in America. This parade of dangerous chemicals changes constantly, and popular ones disappear, while new ones are promoted as the "Magic Answer" to hypertension. One is far better off *doing absolutely nothing* than taking these. They falsely trick the body into lowering pressures, and do not add to quality or length of life. Quite the opposite.

We will not discuss hypotension, or low blood pressure per se, for various reasons. This is very rare compared to high blood pressure. There is almost no research in the international clinical literature on this condition. The bottom line here is that you can cure low blood pressure the very same ways as high blood pressure. Diet, exercise, supplements, hormones, fasting (if possible), no prescription drugs, and ending or limiting any bad habits should cure this in six months or less. If someone has a weak heart, or is very elderly, the results will be much less of course.

America and Japan are the most stressful countries in the world, but this simply does not explain our current epidemic. Happy people have lower blood pressure. Healthy people have lower blood pressure. Happy marriages make for lower blood pressure. Loneliness is strongly associated and many people are lonely, especially the elderly, widowed, and divorced. Happiness and satisfaction with your job or vocation are also factors. Owning a pet, especially a dog, means lower blood pressure. People who go to church regularly and are spiritually minded have lower blood pressure. Psychological issues of all kinds also raise blood pressure. It's not just stress.

Hypertension does not merely mean poor quality of life and early death. Many, many medical conditions are associated with it. Heart disease is the biggest killer of all by far. Hypertension exacerbates any heart or artery problem. Hypertension predisposes one to an endless litany of diseases such as various cancers and diabetes. Some studies have said it is the major cause of erectile dysfunction (ED) in men. Haya Hospital in Spain found a very high incidence of ED in hypertensives. It contributes to Alzheimer's, senility, mental decline, loss of memory, sleep disorders, lack of energy, poor cognition and other problems as we age. At Kuwamizu Hospital in Japan sleep disorders were correlated with hypertension, Metabolic Syndrome, and insulin resistance. The National Institute on Ageing links dementia as directly correlated with higher blood pressure. The Third National Health and Nutrition Survey found that the higher the blood pressure the poorer the cognitive performance in people over 60.

Political correctness tells us there are no differences between the races other than skin color. Scientists, however, know there are countless biological and psychological racial differences. People of African heritage in America, but not in Africa, have epidemic rates of hypertension, diabetes, heart disease. prostate cancer, breast cancer, and other conditions. Latinos in America are more susceptible to insulin resistance and subsequent hypertension, but not in their native countries. All these factors lead to shorter life spans for people of color. To deny racial differences means these people will not get the care and treatment they need, nor the preventive measures to avoid these unnecessary health conditions.

High blood pressure is the most prevalent medical condition on earth, while the causes and cures are all too obvious. This is an *unnecessary* epidemic.

Chapter 2: Diagnostics

How do we diagnose this? How do you know if in fact you really have hypertension or pre-hypertension? What markers are most important? Certainly the most important and basic test is simply one's diastolic and systolic blood pressures. *If you are over 90 diastolic or 140 systolic, these are the accepted cutoff points.* **90/140 is the Magic Number.** Of course, you would really rather be looking at levels of more like 120 over 80. Pre-hypertension occurs when you get to a level near 130 over 85. If you are pre-hypertensive, always remember that an ounce of prevention is worth a pound of cure. Be proactive and do something about it.

There are other important tests. Your blood sugar level is vital here. Know your fasting blood sugar level. *This should be 85 or less.* Do not accept the usual limit of "100 or less," from the medical conglomerate, no matter what your doctor tells you. It is an established fact *that sickness and mortality increase with any blood sugar level over 85.* You can get an inexpensive and accurate home blood sugar meter at the drugstore. The problem here is that some people have a normal blood sugar level, but are still insulin-resistant. If your level is over 85, definitely get a safe, accurate, inexpensive glucose tolerance test (GTT). *The GTT is the Gold Standard.* You test your blood sugar, drink a measured 75 g cup of glucose solution, wait two hours, and test your blood sugar again. It should be under 100, and not merely under 110, as the doctor will tell you. *Anything over 100 indicates insulin resistance.* The GTT is the gold standard here, and is very underutilized. Even if your fasting glucose is 85 or less you really should still get this inexpensive test done. The H1ab test is excellent, and can show your blood sugar average over the past three months. *You should have a level of 4.7 or less.* This equates to a blood glucose level of 85. You really don't need this test unless you are diabetic, pre-diabetic, or suspect you are diabetic. You can find inexpensive H1ab tests on the Internet without a doctor. This three month average is very reliable.

Test your total cholesterol (TC) and triglycerides (TG). HDL (high-density) and LDL (low-density) levels are also useful, but not as necessary. Your TC and TG are far more important. *Your total cholesterol is the best indicator of all for heart and artery disease in general.* Some studies show good correlation of high TC and hypertension, and some don't. You must test your total cholesterol every year. Inexpensive home tests are available on the Internet as well. Your total cholesterol should be about *150 or less*, not 200 or less as you're commonly told. *Mortality and sickness increase with any level over 150*, and especially over 200. American adults test about 240, and this is why heart disease of all kinds is so prevalent. This applies to all types of coronary heart disease. You must keep your level around 150 for optimum health. Yes, this is a practical ideal, and billions of rural Asians and Africans prove it. They have only a fraction of the CHD conditions we do. However, if they move here and adopt the Western diet, they get just as much or more heart and artery disease. *High total cholesterol is basically due to intake of saturated animal fats from red meat, poultry, eggs, and dairy foods.* The best way to keep your cholesterol down is to omit or limit your intake of these. You can eat 10 percent seafood if you like.

High triglycerides are far more important here. Science agrees that triglycerides are a proven indicator of hypertension and CHD in general. Your triglycerides should be *100 or less*. Mortality and sickness increase with any level over 100, especially diabetes and other blood sugar disorders. High triglycerides are one of the very basic signs of hypertension. High levels are generally due to excessive intake of any simple sugars including fruit juice, honey, dried fruit, white sugar, and others. All simple sugars have the same effect, and honey is simply no better than white sugar. High TG is not due to fat intake like cholesterol is. Nearly all vegetarians have excessive intake of simple sugars with resulting high TG levels. Your level must be less than 100. Limit your simple sugar intake and you'll do fine.

If you are over 40, it's a good idea to get your C-reactive protein (CRP) tested. This is an excellent and accurate marker of coronary heart disease (CHD) and chronic inflammation. High CRP is very clearly correlated to high blood pressure, and should be 0.1 to 0.3 mg/dl. The researchers of the world are in agreement that CRP is a reliable marker of blood pressure. Sungkyunkwan University in South Korea found there was a significant positive association between blood pressure and CRP. At the famous Brigham Hospital in Boston they found that CRP levels are associated with the future development of hypertension, which suggests that hypertension is part of an inflammatory disorder. Even children now suffer from high blood pressure. At the University of Wittten in Germany doctors said obese children demonstrated significantly higher levels of CRP compared to non-obese children. The Shenzhen Hospital in China stated, plasma CRP level was positively correlated with glucose tolerance degree in essential hypertension patients.

Homocysteine (Hcys) is also a very accurate marker of CHD events, but is not as strong an indicator of high blood pressure. The evidence here is sometimes conflicting, but the positive ones far outweigh the negative. This is irrelevant in the sense that Hcys is a very basic and vital marker for heart and artery health in general. You should still keep your Hcys level under 10 mmol, and preferably well under 10. You should still get this tested to know the status of your heart and artery health. At Shanxi Hospital in China (*Zhonghua Laonian* 8, 2006) they clearly found, "A positive relationship was found between pulse pressure and homocysteine. This relationship remained after adjustment for classical essential hypertension risk factors". At the Preventive Medical Center in Japan (*Hypertension Research* v 29, 2006) they said, "These data suggest that high plasma homocysteine is associated with increased systemic arterial stiffness, which may enhance blood pressure." At Affiliated Hospital in China (*Shandong Yiyao* v 46, 2006) they found, "In conclusion, the attack of hypertension complicated by ischemic stroke in old patients had a relationship with the increase in plasma homocysteine." They suggested vitamin supplementation instead of drug therapy. At General Hospittal in Taiwan they concluded that hypertensive subjects had higher fasting plasma Hycs concentration insulin resistance. Some studies have found no relationship. This is irrelevant in that Hycs is a proven diagnostic marker for CHD, in general. Even if Hycs is not a completely reliable tool for hypertension, it is a time proven one for over-all heart and artery diseases. This is the bottom line. The famous Framingham Study found (*Hypertension* v 42, 2003) no major relationship. Another review of the Framingham Study (*Clinical Chemistry* v 41, 2003) said it was, "unproven".

Uric acid is very important. Only 15 percent of our blood uric acid is caused by the purines in our food, while 85 percent is endogenous and made by our bodies. Your level should be under 5 mg/dl. Animal foods promote uric acid due to animal proteins and saturated fat. Alcohol definitely promotes uric acid production. Our excessive intake of beef, pork, lamb, chicken, turkey, eggs, dairy products of all kinds, and organ meats causes high blood uric acid levels. You can eat fish and seafood in moderation (10 percent of your diet) if you so choose.

Vegetarians simply don't have this problem. Have you ever heard of a vegetarian with gout or high uric acid levels? Lacto-ovo "vegetarians" who eat diary and/or eggs, yet call themselves "vegetarians" do have higher uric acid levels, even though there are no purines in dairy products or eggs.. High uric acid is associated not only with gout (the most painful form of arthritis), but many other illnesses. You definitely want low uric acid levels. There is no uric acid in plant foods; the problem is caused by the proteins and fats in animal foods. This is why you limit fish and seafood to 10 percent of your diet if you don't want to be a vegetarian.

People in the highest quarter (quartile) of blood uric acid have three times the CHD death rate compared to those in the lowest quarter. People in the highest quartile have over twice the all-cause mortality of those in the lowest quartile. Low uric acid is your ideal, and you can only attain this by avoiding or limiting meat, poultry, and eggs. All dairy foods must go. At Osaka University (*European Journal of Epidemiology* v 18, 2003) the doctors concluded, "These results indicate that high serum uric acid level is closely associated with an increased risk for hypertension, and impaired fasting glucose or Type II diabetes." At the Institute for Cardiology in Poland the doctors there found hypertensive patients showed increased serum uric acid levels and a higher incidence of hyperuricemia. The same results were found in Tottori University in Japan, Shangxi Medical University in China, Hiroshima University in Japan, Baylor College in Texas, and many other hospitals and clinics around the world.

At the University of Verona in Italy (*Metabolism, Clinical and Experimental* v 45, 1996) they found an astounding 88 percent of hypertensive subjects had high blood uric acid. At the Moscow Meditsina Klinicheskaya 79 percent of hypertensives had high uric acid. At the National Cardiovascular Center in Japan (*American Journal of Hyper-tension* v 15, 2002 patients were put on a healthier diet, which caused them to lose weight and lower their uric acid levels. This, of course, resulted in impressive reductions of their systolic and diastolic pressures. The famous Bogalusa Heart Study showed high uric acid levels were clearly and strongly correlated with hypertension, even in children. The most impressive of all is the Framingham Heart Study. This is the longest and largest CHD study in history. The researchers there concluded, "In summary, serum uric acid level was an independent predictor of hypertension incidence..."

Since the kidneys are so central to blood pressure regulation, there are two very important tests that reveal kidney function. Creatinine (not to be confused with the amino acid creatine) is a very good indicator of kidney health. Values vary from lab to lab. If the range is, say, .8 to 1.3 mg/dl for men over 60, and .6 to 1.2 for women over 60, then you want to be right in those narrow ranges. There are no kidney specific supplements, so the answer here is a low-protein diet with no meat, poultry, eggs or dairy, and only 10 percent seafood if you wish. Salt should be moderated, and high salt foods like pickles, salted chips, olives, etc. should be avoided. There is no reason to go on an ultra low salt diet, as explained in Chapter 9: The Low-Sodium Myth. You still must avoid excessive use of table salt.

A good kidney test to use along with creatinine is albumin (protein) in the urine known as microalbuminuria. Albuminurea is highly correlated with arterial pressures. This is called urinary albumin excretion or UAE. It is tested by collecting urine for a period of time such as 8 hours. Any reading more than 15 mcg per minute is considered proof of excessive excretion. There is a spot test where any reading over 30 mcg per liter is evidence of damage. This shows kidney damage and is known as "incipient nephropathy." At the University of Insubria (*American Journal of Hypertension* v 14, 2001) they said, "In conclusion, in never-treated hypertensive patients, microalbuminurea is not only associated with greater myocardial mass (enlarged heart), but is also related with preclinical impairment of LV (left ventricle) diastolic function." At the University of Pisa they found that microalbuminurea accompanied by evidence of sub-clinical inflammation is a strong correlate of metabolic abnormalities in essential hypertension, and identifies a patient subset at very high cardiovascular risk. At Sungkyunkwan University in South Korea they stated albumin and CRP were significantly higher in the hyper-tensive patients. At Brazil's Federal University they saw UAE rate was found to correlate positively with systolic doctor's office blood pressure measurements and ambulatory blood pressure. Kidney prob-lems are caused by excess animal protein in the diet. This generally only comes from meat, poultry, eggs, and dairy consumption. Excess salt intake also stresses the kidneys forcing them to constantly excrete the excess sodium to maintain the vital sodium-to-potassium balance. Hypertension is usually related to weak and damaged kidneys. These are the people who are salt sensitive. It is not sodium chloride that causes their problems, but rather the impaired kidney function that can no longer maintain the sodium homeostasis in the blood. Such people DO need to limit salt intake because their kidneys can't handle the load. This does not mean an obsessive low salt diet with special foods at all, but merely the moderation of added salt to their food. They need to go on a low calorie, low protein diet and fast regularly until their kidneys strengthen and repair themselves.

The liver must be mentioned as well. The SGOT and SGPT, along with bilirubin, are the major indicators. The liver is central to blood sugar production from glycogen. Our livers are harmed by in-take of fats (especially saturated animal fats), alcohol, and most all drugs, especially pharmaceuticals. A routine blood analysis will have these three levels listed along with their ranges.

Chapter 3: Insulin Resistance is the Key

Why do some people raise their blood pressure, and others don't, when subjected to the same life situations? The answer is insulin resistance, more than any other factor. *This includes all blood sugar dysmetabolism in general.* Whenever you study hypertension you find insulin resistance more than any other factor. There is a wealth of information on the action of insulin, blood sugar, metabolic syndrome, and insulin resistance as the basis for hypertension. This chapter will purposely over quote studies to make the point as strongly as possible. You'll see overemphasis and repetition because this is so basic. This entire syndrome is pre-diabetic, and is epidemic in America. Much of this goes undiagnosed, and therefore untreated.

Why are blood sugar problems so epidemic? There are four main causes, but *the main cause is our extreme consumption of simple sugars.* Americans stuff down over 160 pounds of various sugars every year that they don't need at all. It doesn't matter whether it's white sugar, raw sugar, brown sugar, fruit juice, dried fruit, corn syrup, honey, maple syrup, fructose, cane syrup, agave, molasses, or any other simple sugar - they are all basically the same. They all have the same negative effect on our health. Sugar substitutes, even stevia, are just as bad or worse. *Sugar is sugar is sugar.*

Another reason is our severe lack of nutrition, especially minerals. We are all mineral deficient. We are overfed and undernourished. We eat twice the calories we need, but don't get the nutrients we need. Read Chapter 7: The Minerals You Need.

Lack of exercise is the third major reason. Very few people do any physical work anymore. The more exercise the better, whether it is aerobic or resistance. Read Chapter 12: You Must Exercise.

Obesity is the fourth major cause. One third of Americans are obese, and many of the rest are overweight. Obesity is not only strongly and directly related to blood pressure but to all-cause mortality as well. Read Chapter 6: Obesity is Basic.

17

Even in a rural agrarian area such as Nepal a quarter of the adults were hypertensive, and even more had abnormal glucose metabolism according to the University of Nepal in Katmandu. How can rural agrarian people with little stress in their lives have such an epidemic like this?

The entire world's scientific community is in basic agreement that blood sugar dysmetabolism is at the heart of blood pressure conditions. Let's look at some of the countless studies. The University of Verona in Italy found fasting insulin was strongly related to body mass index, waist-to-hip and waist-to-thigh circumference ratios, serum lipids, and blood pressure. The Royal Victoria Hospital in England found insulin clearance was reduced in the hypertensive group. Nerima General Hospital in Japan saw that the most important determinant of systolic and diastolic blood pressures was the plasma insulin concentration. Ichihara College in Japan established that abnormal glucose tolerance (assessed by a 75 g oral GTT) had direct pathophysiological relevance to endothelial dysfunction in moderate hypertensive patients. Sapporo University in Japan (*Hypertension Research* v 18, 1995) reported "The results indicate that 1) insulin sensitivity declines with age, and 2) insulin sensitivity is already diminished in early hypertension. Insulin sensitivity is low in patients with essential hypertension (EH)." Hiroshima University in Japan found that hypertension was positively associated with a significant elevation in BMI, triglycerides, uric acid, fasting glucose, fasting insulin, and 1,2, and 3 hour GTTs, as well as a decrease in HDL.

At Taipei Veterans Hospital in Taiwan it was found that fasting insulin concentrations were significantly associated with systolic and diastolic blood pressures after accounting for sex, BMI, and waist-to-hip ratio. At UCLA they concluded insulin resistance was related to hypertension and blood pressure in subjects without diabetes.

At Middlesex Hospital in England the doctors very wisely suggested that a GTT should be a routine test for anyone over 40 and anyone who suspects a blood sugar issue. *This is true even with a normal fasting blood sugar level.* Much of insulin resistance goes undiagnosed, and the GTT is severely underused. At Joujinkai Hemodialysis Clinic in Japan they stated very clearly that hypertension is caused by metabolic syndrome. Remember that the accepted definition of insulin resistance is much less strict than in the real world, just like the blood sugar, cholesterol, and triglyceride levels. The real world figure here is more like 80 percent. Again, at the same facility they found that insulin resistance seems to have a closer relationship to blood pressure than does plasma insulin.

At Japan Cardiovascular Center it was concluded that insulin resistance, rather than hyperinsulemia, is closely associated to essential hypertension. At Sungkyunkwan University their results showed that insulin resistance, body mass index, and waist circumference are independent risk factors of a high blood pressure in South Koreans. Clearly obesity is 1) strongly correlated with insulin resistance, and 2) a strong factor in hypertension per se. At the Italian Institute Auxologico they found in their subjects that systolic blood pressure correlates significantly with both fasting plasma glucose (FPG) and glucose levels measured 2 hours after an oral glucose ingestion (2-h PG), even after adjustment for age and obesity. Furthermore, lean men with impaired fasting glucose (IFG) had a double multivariate-adjusted risk of hypertension compared to those with normal FPG. At Huddinge Hospital in Sweden they suggested a routine GTT since blood sugar levels are often normal in those with insulin resistance.

Three studies from Poland are clear. At the Academy of Medicine it was found that the mean values of insulin levels were, *in every case*, elevated in patients with essential hypertension. The Tetniczego Academy concluded that patients with hypertension had lower insulin sensitivity. The Endocrinology Clinic found the mean concentration of blood glucose was higher in patients with essential hypertension. Much research has come from China. At First Hospital insulin resistance appeared in essential hypertension patients with impaired glucose tolerance and (or) hyperinsulemia. At the Shandong Hospital doctors said that the levels of fasting glucose, insulin, and total cholesterol in the hypertension group were significantly higher than those of the controls. At Xi'an Medical University it was noted that essential hypertension is correlated with a metabolic disturbance characterized by insulin resistance. At Quingdao Medical College the results suggested that the synthesis and release of insulin were increased in the essential hypertension patients. General Naval Hospital found impaired glucose tolerance, hyperlipidemia, obesity, hyperinsulemia, and insulin resistance in patients with hypertension. At Yangzhou Medical College the patients with hypertension and simple obesity had significantly higher levels of plasma glucose and insulin than normal. At Beijing's Friendship Hospital the doctors concluded that age, sex, BMI, fasting and 2 hour GTT glucose, and insulin levels were all positively related to blood pressure. At First Affiliated Hospital they also suggested using a routine GTT with hypertensives.

How do we cure insulin resistance? Eat a whole grain based diet, with no added sweets or sugars of any kind as much as possible. Limit fruit intake to 10 percent of your diet. Do not eat desserts, dried fruits, or drink fruit juice. Do not use sugar substitutes like stevia or sucralose as studies have shown your body accepts these as they would any simple sugar. In fact, you don't even need sugar in your diet. Read the article *"Fruit Has Almost No Nutrition"* on my website for more information. Fruit is basically sugar (sucrose and fructose), water, and some fiber, with almost no vitamins, minerals, or other nutrients worth mentioning. Eat two meals a day. Fast one day a week. Limit intake of meat, poultry, and eggs if you insist on eating them. Take dairy foods out of your life completely, as all adults of all races are lactose intolerant, and casein is a proven cancer promoter. Take proven supplements like lipoic acid, beta glucan, and CoQ10. Take a good mineral supplement with twenty elements in the amounts you need. Insulin is a basic hormone, and all hormones work harmoniously together in concert as a team. Balance all your other basic hormones, so your insulin will be as effective as possible. Exercise regularly to burn off any excess sugar. *You MUST exercise to cure any blood sugar condition.* You will lose weight without trying while eating all you want if you just do these simple things.

A total program of diet and lifestyle and nothing less.

Chapter 4: Whole Grains

Whole grains are the very basis of your diet. Americans, however, eat a mere 1 percent whole grains of their daily fare. This should be at least 50 percent. Brown rice, oatmeal, polenta, whole wheat and brown rice pasta, whole grain breads, barley, whole wheat couscous, corn meal, buckwheat, rye, and other whole grains should be your staff of life literally. The word "cereal" comes from the Roman goddess Ceres. Man became free from hit or miss survival when he developed agriculture, rather than just hunting and gathering. Grains have been the staple food of nearly all cultures throughout history. This is the difference between cavemen and those who created their own destiny. Studies around the world show that people who eat the most whole grains live the longest and have the best health and least disease. The Okinawans are the ultimate example here. They live the longest and are the healthiest of all cultures with whole grains as their staple.

Let's discuss the basic grains of the world. Rice is the most consumed food on the face of the earth. It is simply incomprehensible that so many people take the time, trouble, effort, and expense to refine these grains and remove the valuable bran and other nutrients. Brown rice should be the center of your meals. You can get brown rice pasta as well. Brown rice flour is very versatile. Sweet brown rice is available, but is meant more for desserts than an entree. Wild rice is really a grass, not a grain. Its distinct flavor makes it better to mix with brown rice. Wheat is the second most consumed food for over six billion people. Bulgur is steamed whole wheat that has been presoaked. You can find whole wheat couscous if you look. Whole wheat and whole grain breads are staple foods. Corn is the third most popular grain. Corn on the cob is a basic food, as are corn kernels. (Frozen corn kernels are perfectly acceptable.) Fine corn flour is known as masa. Most all grits are refined. Course corn meal makes polenta when you add 3 cups of liquid for every cup of meal. There are corn pastas, but they tend to fall apart. Oats are generally only eaten as hot oatmeal for breakfast. Oat flakes go well in multigrain breads. Barley is a fine grain, and can be eaten as an entrée like rice, and not just limited to barley soup. Buckwheat has a distinctive taste and can be mixed with other grains. Rye has a very strong flavor, and is best used in multigrain breads. Millet is a staple in some countries but little used here. It can be used just like rice. Spelt, teff, and quinoa (KEEN-wah) are ancient grains that cost a little more, are very good, but are not well known.

You are dealing with insulin resistance and glycemic control more than anything. A whole grain based diet is the means to control these. At Yonsei University in South Korea (*Atherosclerosis, Thrombosis, and Vascular Biology* v 21, 2001) patients were fed a whole grain based diet for just 16 weeks. Their blood glucose fell an amazing 24 percent, and their insulin levels 14 percent. Lipid peroxidation (oxidized blood fats) fell 28 percent, which means less heart disease. This was done without any other treatments, just better diet. *Diet is the cure for insulin resistance and hypertension.*

At the U.S. Department of Agriculture (*Journal of the American College of Nutrition* v 19, 2000) they reported, "Consumption of, and number of, grains has been reported to control or improve glucose tolerance and reduce insulin resistance. A number of whole grain foods are beneficial in reducing insulin resistance and improvement in glucose tolerance." They suggest eating more whole grains, since Americans eat them as only 1 percent in their diet.

Researchers at Shaheed University in Tehran (*European Journal of Clinical Nutrition* v 59, 2005) studied 827 men and women and concluded, "Whole grain intake is inversely, and refined grain intake is positively, associated with the risk of having metabolic syndrome. Recommendations to increase whole grain intake may reduce this risk."

At world renowned Harvard University (*American Journal of Clinical Nutrition* v 75, 2002) insulin sensitivity was improved greatly with the addition of whole grains to the diet. "Insulin sensitivity may be an important mechanism whereby whole grains reduce the risk of type 2 diabetes and heart disease." They suggested, "People should be encouraged to replace the refined grain foods in their diet, such as white bread and bagels, refined grain breakfast cereals and white rice with whole grain choices." The researchers found that insulin sensitivity improved in a group of obese adults when they ate a diet rich in whole grain foods such as brown rice, oats, barley, and corn. The conclusion was, "Whole grain foods may have favorable effects on insulin sensitivity. These effects may reduce the risk of type 2 diabetes and heart disease." In the *American Journal of Clinical Nutrition* (v 75, 2002), whole grains significantly increased insulin sensitivity and lowered insulin levels. This resulted in lower blood pressure of course. This also from Harvard University, "People should be encouraged to replace the refined-grain foods in their diet, such as white bread and bagels, refined-grain breakfast cereals, and white rice with whole grain choices."

At Simmons College in Boston (*American Journal of Clinical Nutrition* v 76, 2002) they reviewed the Health Professionals Study of over 50,000 men and women for ten years. This covered a half million person years. The more whole grains the people ate the healthier they were, and the lower their blood pressure and the less diabetes. In the same volume of *AJCN* from the U.S. Department of Agriculture (and Harvard and Tufts) almost 3,000 people were studied. Again, the more whole grains they ate the lower their blood pressure, the less heart disease and diabetes. "Increased intakes of whole grains may reduce disease risk by means of favorable effects on metabolic risk factors." Also in the *AJCN* (v. 86, 2007) Harvard did another study and said, "The fiber and nutrients in whole grains help prevent high blood pressure." Each serving of daily whole grains lowered blood pressure a full 4 percent per decade.

Diabetes Care (v 27, 2004) published, "DASH Diet Improves Insulin Sensitivity as Well as Hypertension". The DASH (Dietary Approaches to Stop Hypertension) diet is much better than the standard American diet, and emphasizes whole grains, beans, vegetables, fruits, and low fat dairy products. It is designed to be high in fiber and nutrients, but low in fat and any type of sugar. There have been many studies on the DASH diet. Here, 52 people were put on this regimen and got up to 50 percent improvement in insulin sensitivity, while dramatically lowering blood pressure in six months.

This is certainly going in the right direction especially for the American Diabetes Association. DASH would be a lot better without dairy products of course.

The University of Kuopio in Finland (*American Journal of Clinical Nutrition* v 77, 2003) found that the more whole grains people ate the lower their blood pressure, and the less diabetes they suffered from. "An inverse association between whole grain intake and type 2 diabetes was found." The less whole grains people ate the more antihypertensive drugs they took. This was based on over 4,000 otherwise healthy people without diabetes.

Men and women (*Journal of the American Diabetic Association* v 106, 2006) were given whole grains for 17 weeks to see if this would improve their cardiovascular health. Both their systolic and diastolic pressures were strongly reduced along with mean arterial pressure (MAP). Their total cholesterol, uric acid, blood glucose and other parameters fell as well. *Whole grains are heart healthy.*

At Penn State University (*Science Daily* Feb. 11, 2008) the researchers said, "Consumption of whole grains has been associated with a lower body weight and lower blood pressure." For 12 weeks fifty obese men and women of all ages were asked to eat whole grain foods along with vegetables and fruits. They even ate a little low-fat dairy products, poultry, and meat. Their CRP fell an amazing 38 percent, and their blood pressure fell as well. They lost 8 to 11 pounds while eating all they wanted. Obesity is a big factor in hypertension as we have discussed.

At the University of Minnesota (*Proceedings of the Nutrition Society* v 62, 2003) 160,000 men and women were studied. "There is accumulating evidence that whole grain consumption is associated with a reduced risk of type 2 diabetes, and may improve glucose control." People who ate the most whole grains had the least blood sugar conditions. This involves too many people to argue with.

Make whole grains your main staple. This should be the very basis of you diet. Eat at least 50% whole grains every day.

Chapter 5: Diet, Diet, Diet

Diet is everything. Diet cures disease. Diet cures insulin resistance. Diet lowers blood pressure. All other factors are secondary to what you eat every day. You can lower your blood pressure with diet (and exercise) alone, without any supplements, fasting, or hormones. Without a whole grain based diet, nothing is going to help you very much. Please read my main book *Zen Macrobiotics for Americans.* We eat twice the calories we need; two people could live comfortably on what one American eats every day. This is why we're the fattest nation on earth. Americans eat an astounding 42 percent fat calories. This is nearly all saturated, artery-clogging saturated animal fat. We only need about 8 percent vegetable oils in our food, so this is more than 500 percent of what we need. We also eat twice the protein we need. We also eat an incredible 160 pounds of various sugars every year that we have no need for whatsoever. THIS is the main cause of insulin resistance- extreme intake of simple sugars. Refined grains are another cause. Americans also eat twice the protein they need, which causes high uric acid levels and kidney disease among other problems. Yet, despite gulping down twice the food they need every day, Americans are completely undernourished, and don't get the vital nutrients they need - *overfed and undernourished.* Twice the calories but half the nutrition!

You should eat according to your environment and your genetics. If you are of tropical ancestry living in a tropical area, you can and should eat tropical and subtropical foods like bananas, avocadoes, yams, breadfruit, papayas, mangoes, yucca, boniato, taro, and other tropical foods. If the same person of tropical ancestry moves to, say, Canada they can no longer eat these, as their environment is now temperate despite their genetics. *Genetics and environment.* Nature provides us the right foods if we're in harmony.

Whole grains are your main staple. Whole grains such as brown rice, whole wheat, corn, barley, and oats, should be the very basis of your diet. This is covered in the previous chapter. Beans are very similar to whole grains. Beans and legumes are inexpensive, low in fat, high in protein, high in nutrients, and very filling. A half cup of cooked beans only contains about 120 calories and 2 percent fat calories. By the way, tofu is a heavily refined food with little nutrition, and should only be used occasionally.

Most vegetables can be eaten except the Nightshades. They include potatoes, tomatoes, peppers, and eggplants. These contain the deadly alkaloid solanine (and tomatine in tomatoes). Avoid tropical vegetables unless you are of tropical descent living in a tropical environment. Also limit foods high in oxalic acid like spinach and chard. Americans eat too few green and yellow vegetables.

You should eat local fruits, but only about 10 percent of your diet. Fruits are mostly sugar and water, and have very little nutrition. That's right, there are almost no vitamins, minerals, or other nutrients in fruits. They are a very poor nutrition source. You actually do not need to eat any fruit at all. Take the concept of desserts out of your life. Most Asian cultures do not include desserts as part of their meals. You do not need desserts. Start your meal with a hot delicious hearty soup, instead of having dessert at the end.

Ten percent of your diet can be seafood if you don't want to be a vegetarian and you have no allergy to seafood. You can easily be a vegan on a macrobiotic diet.

Eat soups and salads made from macrobiotic ingredients for variety. Get some cookbooks - be creative.

All dairy foods have to go folks. Milk and dairy foods are absolutely the worst possible choices. This includes the low fat and no fat varieties. Taking lactase tablets such as Lactaid® is also not the answer. Goat, buffalo, camel, zebra, yak, giraffe, or whale milk are all basically the same, as they all contain lactose and casein. There is a universal allergy to lactose or milk sugar. No adult of any race can digest lactose after the age of three. We stop producing the enzyme lactase after that age. Lactose does not merely pass harmlessly thru your digestive system, but causes serious problems. Asians, Africans, American Indians, and other races are hypersensitive to lactose. The milk protein casein is the second reason not to eat dairy products. Casein is proven to promote various cancers, diabetes, coronary heart disease, and other such illnesses. The best discussion of this is found in Colin Campbell's book, *The China Study*. Here he proves beyond any doubt that the intake of animal proteins causes high disease rates and early death. Hard and soft cheeses are almost devoid of lactose, but full of casein and saturated fat. Yogurt is not a health food, and never has been, as it is full of lactose and casein.

Fats and oils should only be 10 to 20 percent of your diet, and from vegetable sources. *20% maximum is the Magic Number here.* There are no "good fats" (other than an omega-3 supplement), and olive oil is not "good for you,"- no matter what you read somewhere. All trans-fats and hydrogenated fats and oils have to be totally avoided. Just read your labels. Labels that read "Trans-Fat Free" can still contain some under the rules. Red meats such as beef, pork, and lamb are too full of saturated fat and cholesterol to be good food choices. No, you don't have to give up red meat completely to lower your blood pressure, but you do have to limit it to 10 percent of your diet. The ideal is to give it up completely, or just eat a four ounce portion occasionally.

Poultry and eggs are among the top ten allergenic foods along with milk and dairy products. Chicken, turkey, duck, quail, goose, pigeon, and pheasant are all the same basically. One large egg has a whopping 250 mg of artery clogging cholesterol. Eating egg whites or egg substitutes is not the answer here either. Just take poultry and eggs out of your diet. Eat turkey on Thanksgiving and Christmas every year if you wish.

The DASH Diet must be mentioned again. Yes, this is a step in the right direction, and certainly easier for people to adapt to than macrobiotics. Whole grains are emphasized as your major food. Vegetables are emphasized as your secondary food. The promoters have no idea that Nightshade foods should be avoided. They also don't understand that tropical vegetables are meant only for tropical people in tropical climates. Fruits are recommended as your third-most important food, when you don't need any fruit at all. Fruit should be limited to 10 percent of your daily food intake. They advise 4-5 servings a day. They also advise 2-3 servings of dairy products. You should have zero dairy foods in your life. They suggest only 2 or fewer servings a day of meat, poultry or fish. One serving would be even better. Most people simply do not want to give up meat, poultry, eggs, or dairy. Beans, legumes, nuts, and seeds are recommended less than one serving a day! Beans and legumes should be eaten every day, and are a major staple second only to whole grains. You certainly don't want to limit them to less than a serving a day. All in all, they suggest you eat a whopping 19 to 24 servings of food a day! You only need two small meals a day. One reason Americans are so sickly is that they eat twice the calories they need. Men only need about 1,800 calories, and women only about 1,200 calories. The DASH Diet just doesn't go far enough, but it is certainly in the right direction.

Terry Shintani (*American Journal of Clinical Nutrition* v 53, 1991) fed obese, sickly native Hawaiians all the natural food they wanted for a mere three weeks. These were low-fat, high-fiber, low-protein meal of taro, poi, yams, breadfruit, fruits, fish and other traditional foods. They didn't even exercise! Their health changed completely in only 21 days, and their blood pressures fell 11.5 mm (systolic) and 8.9 mm (diastolic). That's dramatic!

At Deakin University men ate the DASH Diet for 12 weeks. Their baseline pressures were 129 and 81, and dropped to 124 and 76. Their body weight fell as well, by a whopping 12 pounds just by eating healthier foods. At the University of Calgary they got even better results with the DASH Diet with a reduction of 11.4 and 5.5 mm in systolic and diastolic pressures, in only 60 days. Obese hypertensives at the University of South Carolina went on the DASH Diet and got very impressive reductions of 8.1 and 7.4 mm in their pressures in only 4 weeks. At the University of Tehran 116 patients went on the DASH Diet for six months. Their HDL went up, their LDL went down, along with total cholesterol, systolic (11 mm) and diastolic pressures (7 mm), blood sugar, and body weight. The most comprehensive review was from Boston University listing the various DASH studies. Yes, this works and proves better food choices lower blood pressure. Admittedly, this is a more appealing approach to the masses, since they can include some meat and dairy, and eat lots of calories. It just doesn't go far enough. The Mediterranean Diet will also lower blood pressure, but this has many problems. Meat and dairy, especially cheese, are included. Most of the rice, pasta and bread are white rather than whole grain. Nightshades, especially tomatoes, are daily vegetables for this diet. The best choices of all are the Asian diets in general.

The diet books in print are a disgrace. There is no other way to put it. Suzanne Somers, for example, has been one of the most popular authors, with such abominations as *Eat, Cheat, and Lose Weight*. She is sickly, obese, with breast cancer, but sets herself up as a poster girl for natural health. The high-fat Atkins Diet killed countless people. He finally fell over of chronic congestive heart disease from following his own inane advice. The South Beach Diet is still killing them. The author is on statin drugs for high cholesterol. The "eat right 4 your type series" is simply asinine. The Weight Watchers diet is a bad joke, and expensive to boot. The same is true of the Jenny Craig system. The Zone Diet has almost disappeared; the author has poor health and is chronically overweight. The raw food advocates are all sugar addicts, and have to add cooked grains and other foods when their health fails. Dr. Perricone is still pushing his Mediterranean stupidity. The entire Glycemic Index is too asinine to comment on with their claims that whole grains raise blood sugar.

There are very few authors out there who have any idea what they are talking about. Susan Powter has written two good books *Stop the Insanity* and *Food*; she is very close to macrobiotics. Neal Barnard is a member of the Physicians Committee for Responsible Nutrition, and has written *Turn Off the Fat Genes*, *Live Longer, Live Better, Food for Life*, and *Eat Right, Live Longer*. Terry Shintani is a very sincere man who wrote *The Good Carbohydrate Revolution*, and *The Hawaii Diet*. Robert Pritikin (Nathan Pritikin's son) wrote a half dozen books on eating better. Dean Ornish wrote *Eat More, Weigh Less* and *Program for Reversing Heart Disease*. (He now calls this the *Life Choice* diet.) Gary Null has written *Get Healthy Now, Vegetarian Handbook*, and *Seven Steps to Perfect Health*. George Ohsawa wrote some very brief and simple books on the basic Japanese oriented diet as did Michio Kushi, Herman Aihara, and other macrobiotic authors.

None of the above authors, unfortunately, know anything about proven supplements, natural hormone balance, and fasting. Real macrobiotics (overall view of life) is about life extension and ultimate health, and must include proven supplements, natural hormone balance, vigorous exercise, and regular fasting.

Calorie restriction is an important part of macrobiotics and life extension. Eat as little as possible by eating low calorie foods. Eat as few calories as possible by making better food choices, NOT by going hungry! You can eat fewer calories by choosing whole grains, beans, vegetables, fruits, and seafood. Americans eat twice the calories they need. A man only needs about 1,800 calories a day, and a woman only about 1,200. Just eat two meals a day; you don't need three. Roy Walford is the only one who wrote extensively on the subject of calorie restriction. *The 120-Year Diet* and *Maximum Lifespan* are his best. Science has verified the power of long-term caloric restriction in monkeys and higher primates, and short term in humans. *Calorie restriction is the single most effective method to prolong life.* You do this by making better food choices. You take in fewer calories by eating all the low fat natural foods you want, not trying to go hungry. Eat two meals a day, take your lunch to work, don't eat out often, fast once a week, do a two day fast once a month. *Just make better food choices,* and you can eat all you want.

Fasting one day a week from dinner to dinner is another way to eat less. A two day fast every month adds to this. Don't think that you can't go a mere 24 hours on water, as you'll find the one day fast completely effortless after a few months. You will actually come to looking forward to your one day weekly fast, since you'll feel much lighter and better with no food in your stomach. Short-term fasting is actually pleasurable. Longer-term fasting is more arduous, but also far more rewarding. Authors who have written good fasting books include Paul and Patricia Bragg, Alan Cott, Lee Bueno, Dave Williams, Norbert Kriegisch, and Eve Adamson.

Chapter 6: Obesity is Basic

America is the fattest nation on earth, and literally getting fatter every day. No one out eats us. We eat twice the calories we need, twice the protein we need, eight times the fat we need, and 160 pounds of sugar we don't have any need for. We are the most affluent nation on earth, with the highest standard of living, but this always brings poor health and high disease rates. Obesity is linked to higher rates of basically every medical condition known. (The exception is osteoporosis since the bones must be stronger to support all the extra weight.) One third of American adults are obese, and many of the rest are overweight. Nearly all Americans are out of shape, and get no real exercise. Eighty percent of diabetics are obese. (One in three American children today will grow up diabetic!) Obesity is second only to diet in causing hypertension. We have to keep going back to the fact that high blood pressure is mainly due to insulin resistance, and insulin resistance is pre-diabetes. All of these factors are just aspects of the same basic blood sugar dysmetabolism.

No diet aid works. There are no chemical shortcuts. None of the diet supplements or drugs work. If any of them did, then obesity would be cured, it would be obsolete. You don't lose weight with Magic Diet Supplements. You lose weight by diet and lifestyle, by making better food choices. Dean Ornish's book, *Eat More, Weigh Less* is a good example of this. Terri Shintani's books, *The Hawaii Diet* and *The Good Carbohydrate Revolution* are other fine books. Eat low-fat, high-fiber, natural foods such as whole grains, beans, vegetables, fruits, seafood, soups, and salads. *You can eat all you want and never be hungry.* **The Magic Number here is 20% or less fat calories**. If you eat, say, 8 ounces of salmon at 30 percent fat you must balance this with 8 ounces of brown rice, or 8 ounces of cooked beans. Please read Chapter 20: Calorie Density in my book *Zen Macrobiotics for Americans* for more information. Just 14 ounces of peanuts, or 19 ounces of sirloin steak, have 2,500 calories, most all of them from fat. That's far more than a grown man needs in a whole day. On the other hand, you would need to eat over five pounds of brown rice, over five pounds of pinto beans, or six pounds of cooked oatmeal to get the same amount of calories.

Human clinical studies done at the famous Cornell University (*American Journal of Clinical Nutrition* v 46, 1987) demonstrated this. Women were allowed to eat all they wanted 24 hours a day non-stop, as long as they ate the offered healthy natural foods. All of these had 20 percent or less fat-calories. A control group was allowed 30 percent fat-calorie foods. It really is very easy to limit your fat intake to one fifth of your calories. The first group of women had impressive weight loss in just 30 days while eating all they wanted, 24 hours a day. The second group lost no weight at all. Again, the average American chugs down 42 percent fat, which is nearly all saturated, artery clogging animal fat from meat, poultry, eggs, and dairy. This is just one of many published studies proving that food per se doesn't make you fat - *it's fat that makes you fat.*

The harmfulness of being overweight is agreed upon literally by every scientist in the world. Let's take a quick look at some of the best of the countless studies about obesity. The University of Valencia in Spain said the association between obesity and hypertension has been well documented in most all racial, ethnic, and socio-economic groups. They suggested long term dietary treatment, and reducing calorie intake through better diet, instead of the usual drug regimen. At the Jiangxi Hospital in China they concluded that the BMI (body mass index) has a close correlation with blood pressure and serum lipid level. Hypertension increases dramatically in women after menopause, largely due to the increased hormone imbalance, not lower estradiol and estrone levels. Low progesterone is another factor. At McMaster University in Canada they claimed that the relationship between obesity, hypertension, and insulin resistance is well recognized. At Sahigrenska Hospital in Sweden they concluded that their findings suggest that general and central obesity is independently related to blood pressure.

Since everyone is in agreement about obesity being a major cause of blood pressure problems, the question really is how can we stay slim and healthy without being hungry? *By making better food choices.* That's how. It really is that simple....make better food choices. You can eat all you want, never be hungry, and stay slim and healthy all your life. Just choose healthier foods to eat. Please read my book, *Zen Macrobiotics for Americans*. (The term "macrobiotics" simply means an overall view of life.) The basic thing to understand is that food doesn't make you fat, *it's fat that makes you fat*. Carbohydrates and protein contain only 5 calories per gram, while fat contains a whopping 9 calories. We're going to purposely review some things from Chapter 5: Diet, Diet, Diet for added emphasis.

The first food to go is milk and dairy products of all kinds, even the low fat and no fat ones. All dairy foods contain indigestible allergenic lactose (milk sugar). All adults of all races are allergic to lactose, as they no longer secrete the enzyme lactase. Dairy foods also contain a cancer-promoting amino acid casein. It is easier than you think to drop the dairy habit, and stop listening to ads that say, "Got milk?" Soy, rice, almond, or oat milks are very tasty, and readily available in mainstream grocery chains from various makers in a variety of flavors. You'll come to prefer them over dairy.

Beef, pork, lamb and other red meats need to be eliminated, or very limited to one four-ounce serving a day. Meat is full of saturated fat, animal protein, cholesterol, and calories.

Poultry and eggs also must be omitted, or very limited. Poultry (of all kinds) and eggs are two of the most allergenic of all foods. Many people have unrecognized allergies to them. Poultry is full of fat, cholesterol, and animal protein. A single egg has a whopping 250 mg of artery clogging cholesterol; two eggs have 500 mg.

Americans eat 1 percent whole grains, when at least half their diet should be comprised of whole grains. Whole grains are the staff of life, your main staple, the very basis of your daily fare. Replace white rice with brown, white bread and white pasta with 100 percent whole grain. Eat hot and cold 100 percent whole grain breakfast cereals. Get a good cookbook that emphasizes whole grain recipes.

Hormones have a strong influence on weight and percent body fat. Anyone over the age of 40 has some kind of hormone imbalance, as well as some people under 40. T3, T4, testosterone estradiol, and estrone are especially important to weight management. Read the hormone chapters in *Zen Macrobiotics for Americans*, *The Natural Prostate Cure*, and *No More Horse Estrogen*!

Proven supplements keep your metabolism at peak performance. Please read my book, *The Supplements You Need*. People over 40 should be taking ALC, acidophilus, beta-sitosterol, beta glucan, beta carotene, carnosine, CoQ10, DIM, flax oil, FOS, glutamine, glucosamine, lipoic acid, minerals and vitamins, NAC, PS, quercetin, soy isoflavones, vitamin D, and vitamin E.

The importance of exercise for weight management cannot be overemphasized. You can lose weight simply by taking a half hour brisk walk every day.

Weekly fasting can be a great way to maintain your weight. Just fast on water from dinner to dinner one day a week. You can also add a two day monthly fast.

Never take prescription drugs as they imbalance your system. You'll never be healthy or happy while poisoning yourself with synthetic, toxic prescription chemicals.

Limit any bad habits. Bad habits breed bad habits, and just encourage you to overeat. Success breeds success here.

Obesity doesn't just cause high blood pressure and cardio-vascular disease. Obesity is closely correlated to every known medical condition and illness. *Obesity is a direct cause of all-cause mortality*. There is no disagreement here. The Birmingham Factory Screening Project was one of countless such studies to prove this. Here 2,878 English adults were studied and closely monitored for a full 18 years. This was a costly and rare ongoing study. "In conclusion obesity is a significant influence on blood pressure and all-cause mortality in this large cohort of subjects screened and followed up for 18 years."

Chapter 7: The Minerals You Need

Every disease and known health condition is due in part to mineral deficiency. *We are all mineral deficient* no matter how well we eat- and very few people eat well at all. One of my ten books is titled *The Minerals You Need*. One of the basic causes of hypertension and blood sugar dysmetabolism is mineral deficiency. You are simply not going to get well until you get all the known minerals you need. There are at least 24 known elements we need, and we get enough sodium, potassium, phosphorous, and sulfur in our diets. Yet, there are only ten elements classified scientifically as essential, but we know there are more than twice that many.

In the last twenty years of international published research there are two studies that stand out. Hubert Loyke, at St. Vincents Hospital in Cleveland, wrote extensive articles (*Biological Trace Element Research* v 58, 1997 and v. 85, 2002). He discussed 28 different elements and their effect on blood pressure. At the Medical University in Lodz 23 elements were studied in humans with hypertension (*Klinika Kardiologica* v 8, 2004). In Russia at the Institute of Earth Crust 23 elements were studied in patients with high blood pressure (*Nutrition* v 11, 1995). All of these were very clear about the importance of getting the minerals we need to have normal blood pressure. Research like this is priceless and shows the real cure for any illness is to treat the cause with nutrition, rather than cover it up with toxic chemicals. At the University of Manitoba (*Nutritional Research Reviews* v 14, 2001) both minerals and vitamins to lower blood pressure were studied, rather than toxic drugs. Doctors like these deserve a lot of credit. Nehru University in New Delhi also showed that minerals are the way to treat hypertension rather than drugs (*Biological Trace Element Research* v 34, 1992). Research like this is priceless and shows that the real cure for any illness is to treat the cause with nutrition, rather than cover it up with toxic chemicals.

The real point, which will be repeated over and over, is that we need all the known minerals, not just some of them. Magnesium, calcium, zinc, copper, chromium, selenium, and vanadium have been studied more than any other elements, but it is almost impossible to do studies on the ultra-trace minerals since their effects are so subtle. We need to realize that we need ALL the vital minerals our bodies require, and not just the most "important." Minerals work together as a team in harmony and synergy with each other. The ideal way to get the minerals we need is to find a supplement with all 20 of the ones we know we need. Let's look in detail at the specific elements:

Calcium has a lot of research for blood pressure. This emphasis on calcium is misleading, however, as are the amounts recommended. Europeans in all countries (along with India) have the highest calcium intake in the world from all the dairy products they consume. The only high calcium foods are dairy products, and no one should be eating milk and milk products. Americans and Europeans also have the highest blood pressure (along with the Japanese) of anyone generally. The official RDA of 1,000 mg a day is simply ridiculous, clinically unsupported, and completely contradicted by epidem-iological studies of billions of people. *A realistic intake would be 250 mg* from diet as this is what billions of Asians and Africans take in every day. You could add another 250 mg from supplementation. The usual citrates and carbonates are effective. There is just no reason at all to overdose on calcium. The RDA is simply wrong.

At the Department of Public Health in Japan (*Maguneshumu* v. 10, 1991) hypertension patients were shown to actually have higher blood calcium levels than controls. Healthy Pima Indians were shown (*Journal of the American College of Nutrition* v. 17, 1998) to have lower blood pressure along with lower blood calcium than normal. The real problem with calcium is not intake at all, but rather *absorption.* You need magnesium, boron, silicon, strontium, vitamin D, testosterone, progesterone, and omega-3 fatty acids, among other nutrients, to properly absorb the calcium you eat.

Magnesium deficiency is very common. Plants use magnesium as the core for chlorophyll, as mammals use iron as the core for blood. Eating a whole grain based diet should give you about 400 mg a day, and you can add a supplement of at least 200 mg. Overdosing on magnesium, or any other mineral, is not the answer here at all. The average American probably only gets about 300 mg a day due to the heavily refined foods they eat. One in seven Americans is seriously deficient in blood magnesium. The best source of all is whole grains, but we eat a mere 1 percent whole grains in our diet. Study after study shows low blood magnesium in hypertension patients. Citrates, lactates, and oxides are effective.

Iron deficiency is as common as ever, even with our excessive consumption of red meat. Iron is occasionally found in high levels in hypertension, but this is due to an excretion problem and not excessive intake. Iron retention and lack of excretion fortunately is a rather rare problem. Iron is the "heme" in hemoglobin, and the basic mineral in our blood. You won't be eating red meat, so you won't have to worry about overconsumption. A good supplement will contain the female RDA of 18 mg. The male RDA is only 10 mg. Common sulfates, fumarates, and gluconates are good choices.

Zinc may be either high or low in those with hypertension; there is just no consistency here. Most people do not get the 15 mg RDA they need from the food they eat. Zinc is found in whole grains, beans, nuts, and meats. Deficiency is especially true for the poor, elderly, and alcoholics. There are about 2.5 g of zinc in the human body, half of which is in the muscles. Whole grains and beans are the best sources. Never take in more than 50 mg of zinc daily. The usual citrates, oxides, and sulfates all work well.

Boron is probably *the most deficient mineral in our diet.* There is no official RDA, but 3 mg is the suggested daily intake. It wasn't until 1990 that boron was even accepted as essential! The research is overwhelming here. Our soils and food are very boron deficient. You would think all vitamin and mineral supplements would contain 3 mg of this inexpensive and vital element, but very few do. This proves the megacorporations have huge advertising budgets, but no research departments. Americans probably only take in a mere 1 mg a day. Be sure you get this in your supplement, as boron deficiency is all too common. Citrates or common boric acid are fine here.

Manganese is very important, and the RDA was only recently established at 2 mg. Whole grains are a major source, along with beans, legumes, nuts, and some vegetables. There is an abundance of research about the benefits for our health. A 2 mg supplement is good insurance for such an important element. We only have a total of about 20 mg of manganese in our bodies. That's all, 20 mg. Whole grains, beans, and leafy green vegetables are the best sources. Sulfates and oxides are effective.

Copper also has an RDA of only 2 mg. Americans probably only take in about half this amount. Some people with hypertension have excessive levels, while others are deficient. Whole grains and beans are the best source. Our bodies only contain a total of about 150 mg of this vital element. That's all. Taking 2 mg in your supplement is good insurance. It would take about 15 mg a day for toxicity, which is very unlikely. Citrates, oxides, and gluconates are all very well absorbed.

Silicon is the ignored or "orphan mineral," and almost never found in mineral supplements. More proof that mega-corporations have no research departments, only advertising budgets. There is no RDA set for this, but 10 mg a day is a safe and effective dose. Do not use horsetail as a source. Silica levels in our foods vary so greatly that it is all but impossible to say which foods are good sources. Bone and joint health depend on silica as a basic building block. The science here is most impressive. Plain silica gel (silicic acid) is a good and inexpensive source. You aren't going to find this in supplements except the one mentioned at the end of this chapter. This is one of the two non-metallic elements we need.

Iodine is very important, and the only other non-metallic element we need to supplement. The RDA is a mere 150 mcg. Eating sea vegetables like kelp, nori, and hijiki regularly, as many Asians do, is not a good idea surprisingly. All seaweed contains extreme amounts of iodine. Overdoses of any mineral unbalance your metabolism and are not simply excreted without effect. The most important value here is thyroid metabolism. There are only about 30 mg in our bodies, and three fourths of this is in our thyroid gland. Only 30 mg. Iodine supplements, however, will just not correct low T3 or T4 levels, or any other thyroid problems.

Chromium only recently has an RDA of 120 mcg. This is often deficient in our diet, due to the refining of the grains we eat. It is critical for proper blood sugar metabolism, and deficiency is one of the reasons for such an epidemic. Never exceed an intake of more than 400 mcg. Do not listen to advertisements claiming their form of chromium is the "only effective one". Regular chelates (a non-metal ion bound to a metal ion for better absorbability) are the best sources.

Vanadium was ignored until very recently, and still there is no RDA for it, even though it is now accepted as essential. Taking 1 mg (1,000 mcg) a day is good, but almost no supplements contain this vital mineral. Do not exceed one or two mg a day, as this is toxic at 10 mg. Vanadium has been shown to be critical for blood sugar metabolism. Deficiency is all too common, due to our intake of refined foods. There is now very good science on the importance of vanadium, especially for blood pressure and blood sugar dysmetabolism. Chelates and sulfates are your best choices here.

Molybdenum has an RDA of 75 mcg, but that may not be enough. Be sure to take a supplement here to insure adequate intake. All common salts are good sources, and you will find this in all your supplement formulas. Molybdenum is safe and non-toxic, even though it is a heavy metal. The research is concerned more with soil and plants, rather than animals and humans. Farmers and gardeners commonly use this in their fertilizer and animal feed.

Selenium finally has an official RDA of 70 mcg, but was ignored until very recently. It is very deficient in both our soils and heavily refined foods. Do not exceed a daily intake of more than 200 mcg, as this is a heavy metal and will accumulate in your body. Whole grains are the very best source. Chelates are the most absorbable form of selenium. Be sure to take it with 200 IU of vitamin E, as they are very synergistic and work well together. Studies show that people with low blood selenium suffer from higher disease rates such as cancer, coronary heart disease, and diabetes.

Germanium is a very important ultra-trace element that you will just never find in mineral supplements. Look for the only one in the world that has it. You only need about 100 mcg of ultratrace elements like germanium. Do not exceed this amount, however, as 100 mcg is sufficient. Clinical human blood studies prove this is a vital element we need, but our soils and our food are deficient, and it is not found in supplements. Germanium sesquoxide and chelates are safe, but germanium dioxide is not.

Strontium is another very important trace element with very good science behind it. You won't find it in mineral supplements, but 1 mg (1,000 mcg) is a good dose. Bone and joint health depend on strontium as a building block, as does calcium absorption. No RDA has been set, but science finally recognizes this as essential. Do not confuse it with the radioactive form strontium-90. Chelates and asparates are good choices. Look for the one supplement that has 1,000 mcg.

Nickel is an ignored ultra-trace element; 100 mcg is all you need. Food and blood analysis of animals and humans show this is an essential element, but there is little research on its benefits, or on the problems caused by deficiency. The research is mostly for soil and crops. Nickel is needed in human and animal nutrition. You won't find tin in the mineral supplements on the market either. Regular salts such as chlorides and sulfates are good.

Tin is also ignored as a necessary ultra-trace element. 100 mcg is a good dose. Common food and soil studies prove this is an essential element. Most of the research has been concerned with tin toxicity from industrial pollution, instead of the benefits. Unfortunately, the FDA irrationally limits the dose to 30 mcg. You never find tin in mineral supplements. Human studies have shown low blood tin levels in some illnesses, so we need more research here. Regular salts such as chlorides and sulfates are well absorbed.

Cobalt is never found in mineral supplements, even though it is the basic building block for vitamin B-12. Food and blood studies prove its importance. We are supposed to synthesize our own B-12, but cannot without cobalt in our blood. We probably only take in about 25 mcg or less, but that is enough. This may not sound like much, but we only need to make about 3 mcg of B-12 daily. Taking B-12 orally just doesn't work, so you must take 1 mg of methyl cobalamin. It must be emphasized that sufficient B-12 is just not found in foods, is orally unavailable, and that a cobalt supplement should insure that you synthesize the 3 mcg you need every day.

Cesium is an important ultra-trace mineral, and 100 mcg is all you need. Do not take more than that. Human blood, common food, and soil studies prove how vital this is for our health. You will never find it in mineral supplements. International studies show the importance of cesium in our soil, our food, and our blood. Cesium is vital for humans and animals. Soon science will admit this and set an RDA. Regular salts, especially chloride, work well here.

Rubidium is not an ultra-trace element at all, as our intake is about 1 mg (1,000 mcg). Taking a supplement of 500 mcg is enough, since common rubidium deficiency has not been demonstrated. This is never found in mineral supplements (except one), and very ignored by science. Found abundantly in soil and crops, as well as in animals and humans. The few studies we have are very positive. Brain levels of rubidium fall as we age. This is definitely required in human, animal, and plant nutrition. Rubidium is found in fruits, vegetables, poultry, and seafood. Chloride is a good form to use.

What about *potassium*? Some suggest taking potassium supplements for blood pressure. We get plenty of this in our diets. The National Institute of Health in Framingham showed serum potassium is not related to blood pressure (*American Journal of Hypertension* v 15, 2002) with thousands of patients. Almost no studies find any benefits for potassium supplements.

In the future, we will find other ultra-trace elements are also vital for our health and well being. It is *very* difficult to study these ultra-trace elements, since they occur in such tiny microgram amounts in our food and in our bodies. *Lithium* is essential, but we probably get enough in our daily food. Megadoses of lithium for depression is medical insanity. *Europium* may well be essential, and science will

41

probably decide this in the next decade. *Gallium* is essential, and science has already shown its value in bone metabolism. *Colloidal silver* is a scam, and there is no evidence that silver is needed in human nutrition. *Lanthanum* has considerable research, and is probably vital. *Indium* is claimed to be effective, but studies do not support the Internet ads you see for it. *Neodymium* has shown promise in both animal and human studies. *Thulium* (not thallium) has also shown promise, but only in soil and plant studies so far. *Praseodymium* has some animal and human nutrition research to indicate possible importance. There are other ultra-trace elements that may also be found to be vital. Meanwhile, if you eat whole natural foods and take the twenty elements we need, you'll be fine. There is only one mineral supplement in the world that has all 20 of these vital elements. You can find it on the Internet by simply Googling "mineral supplements." We cannot recommend name brands.

While these good minerals support our health, the "bad" minerals do the opposite. Due to industrial pollution there are elements that build up in our systems, raise our blood pressure, and cause other problems. These include lead, cadmium, aluminum, arsenic, mercury, and thallium. Lead is the most prominent toxic metal for humans (especially for African Americans, but not Africans), with aluminum second. Mercury and cadmium are lesser common toxins, along with arsenic and thallium. The Burns and Allen Research Institute in Los Angeles did an entire study (*Medical Hypotheses* v 59, 2002) showing how common lead toxicity is, and that it is a significant cause of high blood pressure. It is a good idea to get a blood (not hair or urine) test for these toxic metals. Aluminum is the only lightweight toxic element. Alzheimer's is strongly correlated with high blood and brain aluminum levels. Do not use regular baking powder (use sodium based instead), or deodorants with aluminum salts (98% of commercial deodorants). Eating well, calorie restriction, exercise, and weekly fasting, are good ways to lower these toxic metals. Three grams daily of sodium alginate, a seaweed extract, for six to twelve months is a good way to get these metals out of your body. (Just Google "sodium alginate" on the Internet for a source.)

Chapter 8: The Supplements You Need

Supplements are very powerful and effective, but ONLY if you are eating and living well. If you are not eating a good whole grain based, low fat diet no amount of supplements is going to help you very much. If you are under 40, you should not have high blood pressure in the first place. Those under 40 only need about eight supplements. These are beta glucan, a mineral supplement, a vitamin supplement, vitamin E, vitamin D, FOS, acidophilus, and flax oil. L-glutamine can be added to that list. Read my book, *The Supplements You Need*. Most of the following supplements are not directly related to blood pressure, but they are vital for overall health. Treat your whole body, and not merely the pressures of your blood. *Holistic health treats the entire body as a whole*, not just one organ or one condition. The healthier your entire body is, the healthier your cardio-vascular system will be.

If you are over 40, you should be taking about 20 proven supplements, plus any hormones you need. If you don't see a certain supplement mentioned here it is because it is exogenous (temporary), or there is no science behind it, despite its popularity. Lycopene, poliosanol, resveratrol, chondroitin, homeopathic remedies, 5-HTP, spirulina, maca, saw palmetto, MSM, oral SOD, acai, and other such products simply have no value, benefits, or supporting science.

Acetyl-l-carnitine (ALC) is simply a more effective form of the amino acid l-carnitine, and is more absorbable. Take 500 mg a day. You can take 1,000 mg a day for a year for serious problems, or if you are elderly. At the Instituto di Medicina in Italy (*Metabolism* v 49, 2000) patients increased their glucose disposal and utilization simply by taking ALC, with no other changes in their diet or exercise. ALC helps support good brain function, memory, and clear cognition.

Acidophilus is a pro-biotic supplement for all ages. Our digestive systems are generally in poor shape from our diet and life style. Take one with 6 billion units and eight different strains. It must be bought and kept refrigerated like flax (or fish) oil. This is best used with FOS and l-glutamine for better digestion. If you feel your digestion is weak, take all three in both the AM and PM, for one year. Weekly fasting on water for one day every week is important here to give your digestive system a rest 52 times a year. For even better results, join the Young Again international monthly two day fast. *Ninety percent of our immunity comes from our digestive system.* Better digestion equals stronger immunity. It works synergistically with aloe vera, too.

Beta glucan *is the most effective immune enhancer known to science.* Our immunity is central to our health, and only a total program of diet and life style will keep it strong. This is an important supplement for people of all ages. Just take 200 mg a day. You can take 400 mg a day for just one year if you like. Read my booklet, *What is Beta Glucan?*, for more information. All true glucans are equally effective, whether from oats, barley, mushrooms or yeast. This has strong science behind it. Don't pay more than $10 for 60 X 200 mg.

Beta carotene is an important, basic antioxidant, and preferable to vitamin A. Beta carotene is the precursor to vitamin A, and is safer and more effective. With blood sugar dysfunction you need all the known basic antioxidants. Do not take any more than this. A time-proven vitamin, take 10,000 IU daily. Antioxidants are central to curing oxidative stress and inflammation.

Beta-sitosterol is the most effective supplement known for lowering cholesterol and triglycerides. Take 300 mg a day. You can take 600 mg a day for a year if your cholesterol is over 200 mg/dl. The typical American diet only provides about 300 mg. This is literally found in every vegetable you eat, but we eat few green and yellow vegetables. This is also the best single supplement to support good prostate and breast health, and is literally 1,000 times stronger than saw palmetto. There is great science behind plant sterols.

Carnosine is an important supplement for anyone concerned about coronary heart disease. Cardiovascular disease is the biggest killer by far, and CHD health is foremost in importance. Carnosine is ironically only found in meat. You can take 500 to 1,000 mg daily. If you feel your heart and artery system is healthy, this is optional. There are strong studies on this.

CoQ10 is very important for any cardiovascular issue. Take 100 mg and no less. This is not found in your food, and our levels fall as we age. Buy only real Japanese (read the label) biosynthesized CoQ10. Real CoQ10 is ubiquinone. *Do not buy ubiquinol,* as it is much cheaper, but unstable with no shelf life. The best price for 60 capsules is about $25, even from mega-corporations. Take CoQ10 with food or flax oil, as it is oil soluble. Do not listen to any claims of "special delivery systems." There is excellent research on CoQ10 and hypertension, as well as on CHD health in general. There is no reason to take more, unless you have a serious heart condition, in which case you can take 200 mg for one year.

DIM (di-indolyl methane) lowers and normalizes estrogen levels in men and women. This is a much better choice than indole-3-carbinol. You must take 200 mg and no less. "Special delivery systems" are all scams. Just take this with your flax oil or food, as it is oil soluble. You can find 60 capsules of 200 mg for only about $12, if you Google "DIM." If your estradiol and estrone tests are in the low normal range (men or women) you do not need this. Low normal estradiol and estrone (and high normal estriol) are the ideal, based on rural Asian people, vegetarians, and macrobiotics.

Flax oil is the best source of omega-3 fatty acids, and much better than fish oil. *All studies on fish oil would apply equally to flax oil.* These are both the best sources of omega-3s. We have a serious imbalance of omega-6 to omega-3 fatty acids in our blood. Just read Chapter 11: Omega-3 Fatty Acids. The international clinical human evidence for the value of omega-3 fatty acids on blood pressure, insulin metabolism, and CHD health in general is overwhelming. Take 1 or 2 one gram capsules a day, or a half teaspoon of refrigerated "high lignan" liquid (1.5 grams). There is no reason to take more than this. The ideal is freshly ground, refrigerated flax seed, but this is not as practical as capsules or liquid.

FOS (fructooligosaccharides) is an indigestible sugar that feeds the good bacteria in your digestive system, but not the bad bacteria. It is an extract of chicory root or the Terminalia plant. Take it with acidophilus and l-glutamine for good digestion. This is a supplement for all ages. Like glutamine, it is a pre-biotic.

Glutamine is an amino acid that helps keep your digestive system healthy. You should take 1-3 grams a day, as 500 mg capsules or tablets. Take it with acidophilus and FOS to insure good digestion. If you have a more serious digestive issue, buy bulk l-glutamine and take six grams a day for one year. Then, 1-3 grams as maintenance. It has no real taste, and mixes easily with your food, or in soymilk. People under 40 can take this as well.

Glucosamine is a proven nutrient for bone and joint health. Do not waste your money on chondroitin, MSM, hyaluronic acid, and other junk. *Glucosamine does not work by itself.* You must use co-factors such as minerals, vitamins (especially vitamin D), flax oil, and hormones such as progesterone, testosterone, and estriol. It takes time and patience to cure arthritis and other bone and joint conditions, as bone and cartilage grow slowly. Take 500 to 1,000 mg a day.

Lipoic acid is a powerful supplement for blood sugar problems. Take 400 mg of regular lipoic acid. The "R-only" form is an expensive scam; nearly all the research is done on normal R,S-lipoic acid. Please read Chapter 7: Lipoic Acid in my book *The Natural Diabetes Cure*. This is not found in food, so you must supplement it. Insulin resistance is the basis of hypertension, and lipoic acid is vital here as part of a total program of maintaining low blood sugar and insulin levels. Lipoic acid works synergistically with minerals, flax oil, beta glucan, and other proven supplements.

Minerals. Please read Chapter 7: The Minerals You Need. You need at least 20 known elements, and there is only one supplement in the world that has them all. Just search the Internet for "mineral supplements" to find one with 20 elements. People of all ages are mineral-deficient, and need to supplement them. Every medical condition known is due in part to mineral deficiency.

NAC (N-acetyl cysteine) is the best way to raise your antioxidant glutathione level. Surprisingly, this works better than taking glutathione itself. Take 600 mg a day. More and more research keeps showing varied benefits for NAC supplementation, including increased immunity. We have animal studies on NAC and blood pressure, and soon we'll have human studies as well. Glutathione and SOD are your two major antioxidant enzymes.

Phosphatidyl serine (PS) is a relative of lecithin (phosphatidyl choline). It is a basic building block of brain cells. Take this along with ALC and pregnenolone to insure good brain function, memory, clear thought, and cognition. Take 100 mg a day. This is now extracted from soybeans, and is an important supplement to maintain a strong, clear mind as you age.

Quercetin is a borderline antioxidant supplement, since it is basically only found in apples and onions in any quantity. Definitely, take this for at least a year. The science is good, and it is a fine, but optional, one to take in 100 mg doses. Most of the studies are on animals, but more and more good human ones are being done.

Soy isoflavones are a proven supplement with endless science behind them. Flavones are plant pigments, and not "phytoestrogens". (There are no hormones or pro-hormones in any plant.) Just take one having at least 40 mg of mixed genestein and daidzein. If you use soy milk regularly, you don't have to take this. The popular anti-soy propaganda is all from the meat and dairy industries, especially the Weston Price Foundation. Billions of Asians over centuries prove that *soy is good food*. The Okinawans are the healthiest and longest-lived people on earth, and eat the most soy foods of anyone. Isoflavone supplements are the most practical and realistic way to take them.

Superoxide Dismutase (SOD) is the other basic antioxidant enzyme along with glutathione. Our blood and tissue SOD levels fall as we age. Low SOD is clearly correlated with hypertension and CHD conditions in general. It does not absorb well orally, and *all oral SOD supplements you see are scams*. Currently there is no practical way to take SOD, and doctors do not inject it. Exercise, good diet, and natural hormone balance all help to keep your SOD levels high.

Vitamins. There are 13 known vitamins, so just take a good vitamin supplement. You must find one with 1 mg of methyl cobalamin, instead of regular B-12 (cyano cobalamin). Regular B-12 is simply not orally absorbable, so methyl cobalamin is the most effective way to do this. Do NOT take mega-doses of any vitamins, as megadoses of anything just hurt your health. Do not take megadoses of any B-vitamin. People of all ages should take a good 13-vitamin supplement.

Vitamin C can be taken as a 250 mg supplement, but no more than that. This is 400% of the RDA. Megadoses of vitamin C will acidify your normally alkaline blood and make you sickly in the long run. *Do not take more than 250 mg of vitamin C!* The long-term side effects will do more harm than good. Antioxidants are a major part of lowering blood pressure, and vitamin C is one of our basic anti-oxidants. You do not need to supplement this once you are well.

Vitamin D can be taken as a 400 IU supplement, unless you are in the sun regularly. Vitamin D3 is really a hormone, not a vitamin. It cannot be emphasized enough that vitamin D deficiency is epidemic in most all countries. Taking a daily supplement can actually add years to your life. Vitamin D is not found in your food; you can only get it by exposure to the sun. Do not take more than a total of 800 IU (400 IU in your vitamin supplement and an extra 400 IU dose).

Vitamin E can be taken as a 400 IU supplement, but only for a year. 200 IU is enough, and is seven times the RDA. Taking 400 IU long-term thins your blood too much, and inhibits normal coagulation. You can simply take 400 IU every other day if you wish. Be sure to use the natural mixed tocopherols, and not the synthetic single d-alpha. The research on this is overwhelming, and goes back decades. Scientists, for a long time, would not even admit that this was vital for human and animal nutrition

Take these proven supplements for optimal health as part of a total program of diet and lifestyle.

Chapter 9: The Low Sodium Myth

You do not need to go on a low sodium diet. This is the most pervasive myth about curing high blood pressure. The famous Framingham Study proved this beyond any doubt. Salt intake was not related to hypertension (except for people with kidney conditions). The Framingham Study is the longest and largest ongoing study on cardiovascular health ever done. Studies, such as the fine, double-blind one done at the University of Barcelona (*Clinical Science* v 101, 2001), simply could not raise blood pressure in people consuming large amounts of added salt. You do, however, have to moderate your salt intake. There are far too many citations to list on this. That is not to say, however, that you can eat all the added salt you want. The average American is estimated to eat almost nine grams of salt daily. Six grams would be much more reasonable. You simply need to *moderate* the salt in your daily food. Whole grains, beans, vegetables, fruits, and seafood have little sodium. Even beef, pork, poultry, and eggs have less than 100 mg of sodium, generally, per 3.5-ounce serving. *Ninety percent of your sodium intake comes from sodium chloride added to your food.* Processing and salt shakers are the two sources.

There are many pseudo-arguments for the low sodium myth. For example, there is a popular argument that some primitive cultures have a low salt intake along with an absence of hypertension. When they adopt the Western diet, and double their salt intake, they sometimes suffer from high blood pressure. The problem here is that *their entire diet and life style changes!* You can't single out salt when their entire diet and way of life changes completely. There are too many variables to even count in such a situation. It should be mentioned that black people, and other ethnic groups, are far more salt-sensitive, and prone to hypertension and must moderate their salt intake (*Journal of the American College of Nutrition* v 14, 1995). This study also showed that only salt-sensitive people, with weakened kidney function, benefited from low salt diets. Other misleading "salt is bad for you" studies find irrelevant changes in blood pressure (e.g. 128 mm instead of 130 mm), yet claim significant changes due to low salt intake.

Salt intake, basically, does not equate to blood pressure, except in people with kidney conditions who are also "salt-sensitive." Decreasing salt intake does not lower blood pressure. The average American probably takes in about 9 grams of sodium chloride. This comes from processing and your salt shaker. Peanuts, for example, have 5 mg of sodium per (3.5 oz) serving, but peanut butter has over 600 mg! Pork has only about 65 mg per serving, but pork sausage a whopping 1,000 mg! Pickles of various kinds, olives, salted nuts, chips, and popcorn have extreme amounts of salt in them. Such foods can only be eaten in moderation, or better, just avoided.

Again, this is not to say you can just eat all the salt and salted foods you want. It is true that people who eat high amounts of salt (over 12 grams a day) often do show kidney damage and higher blood pressure. It is the kidneys that regulate the sodium level in our blood, and excrete the excess. High salt intake stresses, overworks, and eventually wears out the kidneys. Kidney disease is epidemic in the West generally. The best blood tests for this are creatinine and albumin. Increased overall mortality has also been correlated with eating too much salt. High salt intake has clearly been shown to reduce insulin sensitivity as well. *Moderation in everything.* You should not eat an excessive amount of any food, obviously, and that certainly includes salt. The Japanese eat more salt than anyone on earth. One problem with the traditional Japanese macrobiotic diet is the high salt intake. Pickled vegetables rather than stir-fried vegetables. Salt-pressed salad rather than fresh lettuce. Miso soup every day. High-sodium tamari soy sauce at almost every meal. Gomasio (roasted sesame seeds ground with salt). Natto as a condiment. It all adds up to an overload.

An 11 page study (*Medical Hypotheses* v 63, 2004) with a full 145 references, was very clear about this. If sodium alone raised blood pressure, why don't common sodium salts like citrate and bicarbonate do the same? *They don't.* If sodium was the problem, any edible sodium compound would act just the same as sodium chloride. Again, about ninety percent of our sodium intake comes from the salt shaker and the processed foods we eat. *Food itself contains very little sodium.* On the other hand, severely restricting salt intake can actually cause problems like excessive renin, high angiotensin levels, and sympathetic activity. At the University of Milan (*Circulation* v 106, 2002) hypertensives were given a severely restricted salt diet. The doctors found, "A moderate dietary Na (sodium chloride) restriction triggers a sympathetic activation and a baroflex impairment. Maintenance of the low-Na diet for several weeks does not attenuate these adverse adrenergic and reflex effects." In plain words you need a little added salt in your diet.

Aren't there published studies to prove salt intake raises blood pressure? Well, the closer you look at these studies, the less you see. At Catholic University in South Korea (*Electrolyte & Blood Pressure* v 3, 2005) the doctors made the claim. The actual results showed a slight fall of 1.5 mm in diastolic pressure when people who used excessive salt were put on a low-salt diet. This is not a relevant figure. At the famous Johns Hopkins University (*American Journal of Clinical Nutrition* v 65, 1997) they got a mere 1.2 mm reduction in diastolic pressure by severely restricting salt. They found that weight loss did, in fact, lower their pressures substantially. At Hirosaki University in Japan (*Blood Purification* v 20, 2002) doctors compared two groups of people. One group ate just 2 grams of salt a day, while the second group ate over 21 grams! Such obviously faulty studies like this are prima facie meaningless. Other studies put the patients on better diets and had them exercise. Then they attributed any improvement in blood pressure solely to salt restriction.

It's "salt-sensitive" people, with chronic kidney weakness, who are affected by added salt. This is due to poor kidney function, rather than salt intake. Doctors at St. George's Hospital in London (*Hypertension* v 45, 2004) were very clear about this. "...those who develop high blood pressure have an underlying defect in the ability of the kidney to excrete salt." Japanese doctors (*Nippon Kaisui* v 59, 2005) said, "Salt restriction is only effective in salt-sensitive subjects. Strict salt restriction might be of hazard to health. The policy of universal salt restriction should be avoided." *The real issue with kidneys is protein intake,* not just added salt. Americans eat twice the protein they need, which damages the kidneys, raises blood urea, and causes a whole host of health problems. A macrobiotic diet is very low in protein, and only includes 10% fish and seafood at most. It is very important to stop, or at least limit, eating red meat, poultry, dairy, and eggs due to the high protein content, as well as the high fat content of these foods. High protein diets will kill you.

The low-sodium diet is a myth. *Simply moderate your salt intake, and lower your protein intake.* Moderate the salt you add to your food. Avoid salted snacks, pickles, and olives. Read the labels on all processed foods their sodium content. Salt in moderation is necessary for life. The word "salary" comes from the Latin word for salt, "sal." Roman soldiers were paid in part with salt because of its great value. Salt has been used as currency throughout human history. You'll find the word salt throughout the Bible. We're all familiar with phrases such as, "salt of the earth." Animals naturally gravitate towards a salt block to lick it. The real cause of hypertension, more than anything else is various simple sugars, not salt. Eating sugar raises insulin levels which, in turn, cause salt reabsorption, rather than excretion (*Rinsho Byori* v 55, 2007). Our completely irresponsible intake of 160 pounds of various simple sugars every year is the major cause of blood sugar disorders, and resultant high blood pressure.

What about potassium, since there is a vital potassium to sodium balance in our bodies maintained by our kidneys? Potassium supplements rarely have any benefit, and potassium is sufficient in our food. Doctors at St. George's Hospital (*Hypertension* v 45, 2005) just got no benefit from giving people 2,300 mg potassium supplements. You would have to take large 1,000 mg, or more, potassium supplements to have any possible effect here. The best potassium source is various fruits. Still, you should limit fruit intake to 10% of your diet or less. You really don't even need to eat any fruit, since it is so low in nutrition. Cooked beans have very high levels of 400 to 500 mg a cup. Cooked brown rice, for example, has about 137 mg per cup. Men take in about 3,000 mg of potassium a day, and women about 2,500 a day. What about the salt substitutes made of both sodium and potassium chlorides? They are expensive, taste metallic, and are just not necessary. In Brazil (*Revista de Nutricao* v 18, 2005) such substitutes were given to people with no benefit at all.

Chapter 10: Temporary Supplements

Endogenous supplements are ones that exist naturally in our bodies and/or our daily food. These include all the ones mentioned in the previous chapter. Exogenous supplements are ones that do not exist naturally in our bodies or our daily food. This includes fruit pectin, ellagic acid, aloe vera, and curcumin. We are also going to discuss temporary endogenous supplements like taurine and TMG. All of these can be taken for six to twelve months only, and then discontinued. Exogenous supplements should be temporary.

Fruit pectin from citrus or apples, taken 3 grams a day (6 X 500 mg), is a very proven supplement for lowering blood fats. You can also use other plant polysaccharides such as guar gum, glucomannon (konjac root), and sodium alginate (from seaweed). Avoid "modified" citrus pectin, which is an expensive fraud. The value of guar gum for lowering blood pressure, insulin, and blood sugar was proven at Royal Adelaide Hospital in 2003.

Ellagic acid is found in black walnut hulls and other plants, such as Terminalia chebula. Make sure the label states that each capsule contains at least 100 mg of ACTUAL ellagic acid. Avoid overpriced raspberry seed products. It will not lower your blood pressure per se, but is a proven herbal supplement that will help your general health and make you more resistant to cancer and other malignancies. Avoid overpriced raspberry seed products.

Aloe vera is a time-proven remedy especially for our digestion and liver functions. Take two capsules of 100 mg 200:1 extract. This equals 40 grams of fresh aloe gel. (Aloe gel is 99.5% water.) It works well with acidophilus, FOS, and l-glutamine.

Taurine is endogenous, and is in your daily food. It has value for diabetes and hypertension. Both conditions often show low blood levels. It still should only be taken for a year in 1 to 2 gram doses. The science behind taurine and diabetes is strong. In 2004, an extensive review of the literature with 114 references at the University of Sassari in Italy was done. It demonstrated good benefits in treating diabetes and insulin resistance.

Curcumin is a well studied and time proven antioxidant from the tumeric root. It is exogenous, so some people will not be helped by taking it. You need all the antioxidants you can take when treating hypertension and insulin resistance, and this is a good one.

TMG (trimethylglycine) is the most powerful and effective liver rejuvenator known to science. Take 3 g (6 X 500 mg) for six to twelve months. You can take 1 g (2 X 500 mg) for the rest of your life if you want which will help keep your homocysteine level low. Read the *Rejuvenate Your Liver* article found at my website.

Sodium alginate from seaweed is a proven way to reduce cholesterol and remove heavy metals like lead, cadmium, and mercury, from your blood. Just take 3 grams (6 X 500 mg) for six months. Google this on the Internet as it can be hard to find.

What about well advertised supplements that are supposed to work to lower blood pressure? Most of these are simply advertising promotions for profit, and not effective at all. Arginine is useless no matter what you read somewhere. Theoretically, arginine is the precursor for nitrous oxide (NO). The only "studies" use insane overdoses either orally or by infusion (drip injections) to get any effects. Thirty years of published research fails to show any value here for supplementation. Bitter Melon (Momordica) just has no science behind it. Gymnema sylvestre is heavily promoted, but where are the studies? Lots of advertisements, certainly. Fenugreek seed also has advertisements instead of studies. Nopal cactus just has no proof of effectiveness. Cinnamon extract is also heavily promoted for blood sugar problems, but there are just no human studies to back this. Temporary supplements are not even necessary, but can certainly speed your healing. Just remember they are temporary.

Chapter 11: Omega-3 Fatty Acids

Omega-3 fatty acids are so important they deserve a chapter of their own. These are also known as alpha linolenic acids (ALAs), as opposed to alpha linoleic acids (LA). Linolenic versus linoleic. Another name is N-3 fatty acids. Do not get confused by all the talk regarding EPA and DHA. If you take flax or fish oil, you will naturally convert these into EPA (eicosapentanenoic acid) and DHA (docohexanoic acid) as needed. *We eat far too many omega-6 fatty acids, and far too few omega-3s.* One reason is that we don't eat a natural foods diet. Another reason is omega-3s are not common in most foods in any quantity. It is really difficult to get omega-3s in your daily food. Grass-fed beef has omega-3s, but is full of saturated fat and cholesterol. Fatty fish have omega-3s, but are 30 percent fat calories. You shouldn't be eating high-calorie, high-fat fish like salmon and tuna every day anyway. The best sources are fish oil and flax oil. Salba (chia seed) and hemp seed are also good sources, but are expensive and hard to find. *Flax oil, is by far, the best choice, and is much preferable to fish oils.* Flax has twice the omega-3 content of fish. Flax oil is less subject to oxidation by light, heat, and oxygen. Oxidation produces toxic lipid peroxides, which we call rancidity. Flax oil is also much less expensive than fish oil, and it is easier to find refrigerated brands. Flax oil has a pleasant nutty taste, whereas fish oil must be taken in a softgel capsule. Fish oils contain dangerous arachidonic acid. Blood levels of this are correlated with various diseases. It would take 3.2 pounds of fresh salmon to equal the omega-3 content of just four tablespoons of flax oil. Flax is the best possible source of valuable plant lignans, which are an important, but deficient, part of our diet. We get very few vital lignans in our food.

Plant sources of supplements are always best when available, since a plant based diet is healthiest. Do not use expensive borage, black currant, or primrose oils, as they all have lower levels of omega-3s. Most of the studies on omega-3s use fish oil, but *all of these studies would equally apply to flax.* Any study that used fish oil would have gotten even better results with flax oil, especially since flax oil contains more omega-3s per gram. Whether you choose fish oil or flax oil, you must buy it and keep it refrigerated. Both have very short shelf lives, and *must be kept under refrigeration.* At room temperature they soon turn rancid, and then have lots of harmful free radicals. Omega-3 fatty acid supplements are vital, not only to a program of treating hypertension, but treating all forms of coronary heart conditions. *Omega-3s are heart and artery healthy!* Coronary heart disease is the biggest killer of all by far. Whether you are concerned about high cholesterol, triglycerides, C-reactive protein, homocysteine, heart attack, stroke, or any other heart and artery related problem, you must take flax oil. You can take 3-4 grams the first year if you want, especially if you are elderly or in bad health. Then, 1-2 grams should be enough. You can also use a half teaspoon (1.5 grams) of high-lignan liquid flax oil. There are only 9 calories in every gram of fish or flax oil, so this does not add to your caloric or fat intake. This is a supplement for people of all ages, including children. It is one of only eight supplements people under 40 need (along with vitamins, minerals, acidophilus, FOS, beta glucan, vitamin D, and vitamin E). You can also give this to your pets. The published studies on omega-3 supplementation are overwhelming.

A very nice review from the University of Iowa (*Current Opinion in Lipidology* v 7, 1996), "N-3 Fatty Acids and Hypertension," was most convincing. It was substantiated by 37 references. They clearly stated, "N-3 fatty acid supplementation reduced blood pressure in patients with essential hypertension." Some of the studies reviewed found omega-3 supplementation made hypertension drugs more effective. This is not recommended at all, since you should do this naturally *without any drugs.* Other studies found heart transplant patients on anti-rejection drugs fared better by taking omega-3s. They also found omega-3s caused vasorelaxation to expand the blood vessels and allow better blood flow.

A very long 14 page review with 96 references was published in *Annals of the NY Academy of Sciences* (v 827, 1997). This is a highly sophisticated article written in very technical language, and meant for professionals. The bottom line, however, is that omega-3 supplementation lowers blood pressure, and is good for overall heart and artery health. They point out that both fish and flax oils are the best sources of omega-3s with flax oil containing the most, at about 50%. They also showed omega-3s help prevent the development of proteinuria (high protein in the blood, especially albumin, from kidney dysfunction). "Reduction of dietary fat, particularly saturated fat, is a key strategy for preventing cardiovascular disease, but it is unlikely to lower blood pressure unless accompanied by weight loss." Then, they emphasize the need for high blood omega-3 levels to keep blood pressure down.

At the University of Tromso (*Annals of Internal Medicine* v 123, 1995) men and women were given expensive DHA and EPA in a classic double blind, placebo study. It would have been more effective to give them inexpensive flax oil. Both diastolic and systolic pressures were lowered significantly, with no change in diet, life style, or exercise. Both triglycerides and low-density (LDL) cholesterol levels also fell significantly. At the University of Trondheim (*16th Scandinavian Symposium on Lipids*, 1991) people were given omega-3 fatty acid supplements. Their blood pressure fell significantly with no other treatments.

At the University of Florence (*Thrombosis Research* v 91, 1998) they stated clearly, "Dietary n-3 polyunsaturated fatty acids can lower blood pressure in humans." Here healthy controls were compared to hypertensives with very good results in only 60 days. At Yokosuka Research Group in Japan (*Journal of Oleo Science* v 56, 2007) they said, "These results suggest that ALA (alpha linolenic acid) has an antihypertensive effect with no adverse effect in subjects with high-normal blood pressure and mild hypertension." At Shimane Medical University in Japan they found, "Increased dietary n-3 PUFA intakes from marine fish and plants may modify the blood pressure and risk factors for CVD and decrease the incidence of CVD."

At Lok Nayak Hospital in India (*Indian Journal of Clinical Biochemistry* v 20, 2005) 100 patients were given flax oil supplements for only 4 weeks. "A significant reduction of fasting plasma insulin levels in both groups was observed (29.0% and 22.8%) as well as serum cholesterol, triglyceride, and LDL, while HDL rose 8% in both groups." This kind of dramatic effect with flax oil alone is nothing less than amazing. They recommended routine flax supplementation, and curtailment of omega-6 intake for hypertension.

At the Barzilai Medical Center in Israel omega-3s were given to hypertensives. "Dietary supplementation with n-3 PUFA decreases blood pressure and serum triglycerides. In both non-diabetics and diabetics, similar significant decreases in blood pressure were achieved with no other intervention. At the University of Trondheim they said, "The results therefore indicate that long-chain n-3 fatty acids probably have the same (positive) effect on blood pressure irrespectively of whether they are taken as fish oil or part of the normal Norwegian diet."

A thorough review (*Omega-3 Fatty Acids*- Drevon 1993) with 18 references went into great detail on the mechanisms for the blood pressure lowering effect of omega-3 fatty acids. The University of Colorado (*Journal of Hypertension* 19, 2001) said omega-3 supplements enhanced insulin resistance. At Weizmann Institute in Israel (*Journal of Clinical and Basic Cardiology* v 5, 2002) people given an omega-3 supplement, and a diet low in omega-6s, benefited greatly. "In the n-3 group we observed a significant decrease of serum cholesterol, LDL, triglyerides, and insulin. Hypertension, which was positively correlated to hyperinsulemia, decreased significantly, especially the systolic." The Institute of Military Hygeine in China (*Yingyang Xuebao* v 14, 1992) gave EPA and DHA to hypertensives for only 10 weeks. "In vitro thrombosis was remarkably inhibited in subjects, and systolic and diastolic blood pressure were markedly lowered". No other treatment but omega-3 supplementation.

The most important study of all (*British Journal of Diabetes* v 8, 2008) showed simply that blood levels of omega-3 fatty acids were clearly correlated with all cause mortality! The higher the level of omega-3s in your body the longer you'll live and the healthier you'll be. This shows just how important omega-3 supplements are.

This is a supplement for people of all ages. Pets, too.

Chapter 12: You Must Exercise

You can literally cure cancer while sitting on the couch watching television all day. Of course, it is always better to exercise, and your healing will go much better and much faster if you do exercise. Really vigorous exercise is best, but just walking a half hour a day is all you really need.

With hypertension, insulin resistance, and diabetes to get well you MUST exercise. There is no way around this. *You must exercise to get well.* Lack of exercise is a major cause of high blood pressure. In rural agrarian societies, one reason hypertension is so rare is due to the great amount of physical work required just to survive and eat. Exercise is so powerful and so effective that some people can cure their hypertension with just vigorous exercise, and no other change in diet or life style. That is not the sermon in this book at all. This is said simply to stress how vital regular daily exercise is to maintaining normal blood pressure levels.

The published clinical studies are overwhelming here. Exercise lowers both systolic and diastolic pressures very dramatically, but does much more than that. It improves many biological diagnostic parameters as well as we'll see in the following studies. At the University of Tennessee (*Preventive Medicine* v 37, 2003) doctors simply had the patients walk every day, with no other changes in their life styles. For eight weeks they simply walked a lot every day. Their blood pressure fell dramatically. At Kyushi University in Japan (*Metabolism, Clinical & Experimental* v. 51, 2002) diabetic hypertensive men used an exercise bike every day. It's harder to lower blood pressure in diabetics because of their generally poor physical condition. They were given glucose tolerance tests (GTT) that showed improved insulin resistance, as well as lowered both systolic and diastolic pressures with no other lifestyle changes. Beta endorphins are the "feel good hormone" that fill our opioid receptors. Exercise raises beta endorphin levels, and makes us feel good naturally. Male hypertensives at the Second Military Medical University in China (*Shanghai Yixue* v 17, 1994) were found to be low in beta endorphins. Two weeks of mild exercise raised their beta endorphin levels, lowered their blood pressure and the men had a greater feeling of well being with no other life style changes.

At St. Thomas Hospital in London (*Circulation* v 101, 2000) male hypertensives were found to have insulin resistance as well as high total cholesterol levels. "Changes in diastolic blood pressure during gentle exercise are strongly associated with serum concentrations of total cholesterol and insulin resistance. This may contribute to development of hypertensive complications in dyslipidemic and/or insulin resistant patients." Notice this was merely "gentle exercise," and not rigorous at all. Russian doctors (*Eksperimental'naya Meditsina* v 26, 1991) found hypertensives had decreased exercise tolerance and high blood lactate levels. Regular exercise gave them a greater ability to exercise longer and dispose of excess lactic acid. Exercise reduces hyper levels of lactic acid in the blood. This builds up as hypertension reduces the body's ability to dispose of it.

A really thorough review, "Antihypertensive Mechanism of Exercise," was done at Fukuoka University in Japan (*Journal of Hypertension* v 11, 1993) complete with 69 references. The urban Japanese (not the rural) have the highest blood pressure in the world. Here, studies around the world were collected. The doctors were primarily interested in understanding exactly how exercise lowers blood pressure, and which mechanisms were responsible. They studied such things as noepinephrine, kallikrein, prostaglandin E, natriuretic peptide, dopamine and ouabain. This gets pretty technical, but the bottom line is that exercise works well, and we don't need to worry about the hows and whys. After reading such a thorough and well documented review, there is no doubt left as to how effective and necessary any kind of exercise is.

At Katedra i Klinika Kardiology in Poland (*Polskie Archiwum Medycyny Wewnetrznej* v 104, 2000) men and women with hypertension were found to have hyper leptin levels. They found, "The moderate, short-term exercise decreases serum leptin levels in the hypertensive patients." Here, exercise was found not only to lower blood pressure, but leptin levels as well. At the Medical University of

Warsaw (*Journal of Human Hypertension* v 12, 1998) hypertensive men were given a daily exercise program. *One single bout of exercise lowered their blood pressure significantly.* This phenomenon has been found in other studies as well. They did a 20-minute session daily on an exercise-bicycle (ergometer). The doctors concluded, "Long lasting antihypertensive effect of a single dynamic exercise in hypertensives suggests that moderate exercise may be applied as an effective physiological procedure to reduce elevated arterial blood pressure in mild hypertension." Notice the term, "long lasting."

At Computense University (*Antioxidants* 7, 2005) they strongly link oxidative stress and inflammation to hypertension. Exercise is very powerful for reducing both oxidative stress and inflammation. They show that exercise is a vital part of any blood pressure lowering program. At Ohio University (*Comparative Bio-chemistry* v 133C, 2002) the doctors also found that exercise improved antioxidant levels and reduced oxidative stress. This led to lower blood pressure with no other changes in diet or life style. At Taipei Medical University (*Clinical and Experimental Hypertension* v 24, 2002) "Moderate intensity regular exercise training in these patients reduces blood pressure." Here, just 12 weeks of using a treadmill reduced systolic pressure a whopping 18 mm with no change in diet. An 18 mm drop is simply amazing. Total cholesterol, LDL, and triglycerides were reduced, and HDL raised significantly. At the University of Naples (*Journal of Human Hypertension* v 17, 2003) more work was done in this area. "The results demonstrate that exercise is associated with enhanced blood nitrosation, and suggest that the ascorbate, or urate, levels increase to limit oxidative damage." In plain words, exercise greatly improved antioxidant function, and oxidative stress was reduced remarkably. They measured six different antioxidant levels in their blood and found all of them to rise after a mild exercise program.

We discussed that insulin sensitivity is at the heart of rising blood pressure. Exercise improves insulin sensitivity greatly. At the University of Michigan (*Metabolism, Clinical and Experimental* v 53, 2004) this was proven with elderly men and women. Older people are much harder to treat. "In conclusion, a 4-month resistance training program significantly increased insulin-mediated glucose disposal and lean body mass...in older hypertensive subjects." At the Laval University (*Circulation* v 108, 2003) doctors noted that two cause of hypertension are reduced glycogen (stored source of blood sugar) synthesis and insulin sensitivity. Mild exercise of any kind raises both very effectively.

At the University of Tsukuba (*Hypertension Research* v. 27, 2004) two separate studies were published. In the first, postmenopausal women did low intensity aerobic cycle-exercise for 12 weeks. Their blood pressure fell significantly. In the second, more elderly women did moderate cycle exercise. Their nitric oxide (NOx) blood levels rose while their blood pressure fell. NOx is very important to keeping blood pressure low, and falls as we age. In the same journal a year later (v. 28) they verified the positive effect of exercise on NOx. They also found their superoxide dismutase (SOD) levels rose as well. "Life style modification is recommended as a non-pharmacological approach to treatment of hypertension" they said. The urban Japanese have the highest blood pressure in the world despite their generally good diet. More and more they adopt the Western ways of high-sugar and high-fat refined foods and suffer the consequences.

At Kansai Medical University (*Clinical and Experimental Hypertension* v 19, 1997) people with hypertension exercised for three months. Of course their blood pressure fell, but other sophisticated blood parameters were very much improved as well.

Exercise is simply good for your entire health. When you exercise everything in your body improves in both overt and subtle ways. *You must exercise to lower your blood pressure.* There is no way around this. You can do aerobic or resistance and you can do low intensity. Join a gym if you can or put equipment in your home. Or you can just take a brisk walk every day. "The sovereign invigorator of the body is exercise and, of all the exercises, walking is the best." – Thomas Jefferson. Do what you enjoy best.

Chapter 13: *Your Basic Hormones*

Maintaining a youthful hormone level is a basic part of real macrobiotics, natural health, longevity, and life extension. Almost no doctors on the face of the earth have any idea what they are doing here. That includes endocrinologists, naturopaths, holistic physicians, and life extension specialists. You have to depend on yourself, and not try to pawn the responsibility off on some doctor who doesn't know what he's doing. They are just not educated about your basic hormones, how to measure them, or how to naturally balance them.

Hormones, like minerals, work together as a team harmoniously and synergistically in concert. We want to have all of our 14 basic hormones at youthful levels as much as possible. We need to go far beyond merely balancing insulin and blood sugar, as all our hormones work together and support each other. Let's look at the basic fourteen:

Insulin
Testosterone
Androstenedione
DHEA
Melatonin
Pregnenolone
T3
T4
Growth Hormone
Estradiol
Estrone
Estriol
Progesterone
Cortisol
(Cholesterol)

With hypertension, the most important hormone we need to deal with is insulin. Measuring insulin directly is not the best way to go surprisingly. We will learn much more by measuring fasting blood sugar and blood sugar response (GTT). If fasting sugar is over 85

63

mg/dl then a glucose tolerance test (GTT) is called for. This is the gold standard, and tells you how effectively your insulin is reacting to the cells in your body. The GTT reveals insulin resistance better than any other test. It should be routine for anyone over 40.

Insulin levels do not reveal as much as insulin *response*. Know your blood glucose. *Your fasting blood sugar should be 85 or less.* Please remember that figure - 85 or less. Do not let the doctor tell you that higher values of, "100 or less" are all right. A one-draw, two-hour glucose tolerance test (GTT) is the best test of all here. This tells you insulin response, and not just insulin levels. You drink a 75 g cup of glucose solution, wait two hours, and have your blood drawn and tested. You want a level of about 100 after the two hours, not any higher. Many people have normal blood sugar levels, but are still insulin resistant. The GTT is accurate, inexpensive and very worth doing. Insulin resistance is the basis of most hypertension,

Testosterone is the basic androgen along with DHEA and androstenedione. Women have only one tenth the amount, but it is vital to their health. Please read my book *Testosterone Is Your Friend*; *A Book for Men and Women.* Men cannot have hyper levels, as they cannot overproduce it. Even if they over supplement it they just make estrogens. Hyper levels in women can only be lowered by diet, exercise, and life style, along with balancing the other hormones. Testosterone is very influential in diabetes and insulin resistance. Hypertensive men are often deficient, while women are often excessive. 90 percent of normal, healthy men over 50 need supplementation anyway. That's right, 9 out of 10 men over the age of 50 are testosterone deficient and should raise their levels.

Doctors are clueless as to measuring and administering testosterone. They also have no idea how important this is to female health. Injections are completely wrong. It cannot be taken orally. DMSO solutions are not legal, although you can make them yourself. Transdermal creams and gels only deliver about 20 percent into the blood and the rest is wasted. The very best way is to use a salt (such as enanthate) sublingually (under your tongue) in vegetable oil. Natural testosterone tastes terrible! Sublingual salts are the best way.

There are a wealth of studies showing male hypertensives are low in testosterone. There is little research on women here. Women who prove to be low can supplement with 150 mcg of testosterone in their blood. Women who have an excessive level can only lower it with a program of diet and life style. There are no safe drugs to lower testosterone in women. Any man or woman over 40 should test their *free* testosterone level and make sure it is at a youthful level. The most famous study was done at the University of Tromso with 1,548 men (*European Journal of Endocrinology* v 150, 2004). "The results of the present study are consistent with the hypothesis that lower levels of testosterone in men are associated with higher blood pressure." They pointed out that this is usually mediated by obesity.

Androstenedione (and androstenediol) is the direct precursor to testosterone. The blood level generally parallels that of testosterone. Men don't need to measure this generally, and women only need to measure this if they have high testosterone or suspect androgenicity. Using androstenedione, androstenediol, or their analogs is not a good way to raise testosterone, and it is now classified as a prescription-only drug.

DHEA is the other major androgen. It is known as the "life extension hormone," for good reason. Youthful levels are strongly correlated with good health and long life. There are countless published international human studies showing how vital this is. Dramatic results are found with proper supplementation. In men and women this is often deficient after the age of 40. In women of any age DHEA can also be excessive, as well as deficient. This condition is called androgenicity, and high testosterone and androstenedione are often found as well. Teenagers generally have very high levels, but it is not reasonable to try and match such youthful levels. Look for the level you had at about age 30. You never, never take DHEA without prior blood or saliva testing to know your level. Men who prove low can take 25 mg, and women who are low can take 12.5 mg (half-tablets). DHEA, like pregnenolone, is only about 10 percent absorbed when taken orally. The only way to lower excessive levels is by diet, exercise, and life style, as well as by balancing your other hormones.

Melatonin is a powerful antioxidant hormone. People don't understand how important and powerful it really is. It is a very under-rated hormone, and science discovers new benefits for it every month. Our levels fall from the time we reach twenty, and almost disappear by the time we're seventy. Most everyone over the age of 40 can and should take this. Take melatonin at night only, and never during the day. The science about melatonin grows all the time, and now it is being used to both to prevent and treat cancers of various kinds. Fortunately we now have both animal and human studies to demonstrate just how important melatonin is in maintaining healthy blood pressure levels. Who else is going to cite studies to show you the value of taking melatonin for hypertension?

At the Netherlands Institute for Brain Research (*Hypertension* v 43, 2004) male hypertensives were given 2.5 mg melatonin every night for only three weeks. This was a classic double-blind, placebo-controlled study. "Repeated melatonin intake reduced systolic and diastolic blood pressure...and also improved sleep." At Policlinico di Modena (*American Journal of Hypertension* v. 18, 2005) women were given melatonin for just three weeks in a randomized, crossover, double-blind study. "These data indicate that prolonged administration of melatonin may improve the day-night rhythm of blood pressure, particularly in women with a blunted nocturnal decline." At the Cincinnatti College of Medicine (*Journal of Pineal Research* v 36, 2004) type 1 diabetic hypertensive adolescents (average age only sixteen) were given 10 mg of melatonin for a week. These poor children had high blood pressure in addition to type 1 diabetes. Their blood pressure improved in only a week. The fact you can successfully treat children with melatonin, is nothing less than amazing. At the Zabreze Biochemical Clinic men and women hypertensives, with an average age of forty-two, were given melatonin. One-third had severe, one-third were moderate, and one-third were healthy. "Results of our studies seem to confirm the concept that decreased melatonin secretion can be one of the causes of hypertension."

Pregnenolone is the forgotten, or "orphan," hormone because so little work has been done studying it in clinics around the world. It is known as the "grandmother hormone," since the rest of the sex hormones are derived from it. This is THE most important brain, memory, and cognition hormone, yet there is little research being done even today. It is best used with PS (phosphatidyl serine) and ALC (acetyl-l-carnitine). There are no studies on the relation of pregnenolone levels to blood pressure for the simple reason there is hardly any research at all on pregnenolone. Youthful levels are necessary for total hormone balance. Pregnenolone falls in men and women at about age forty, and then levels off, and stays low the rest of one's life. In 2009 some lab should finally offer a reliable saliva home test. You can get a blood test from a doctor for about $100, plus the office visit. Generally, men over forty can safely take fifty milligrams, and women 25 milligrams. As with DHEA, men have much higher levels of this. Only about 10 percent of pregnenolone (and DHEA) is absorbed when taken orally. This is the only practical way to take them however. Since all your hormones work together harmoniously in concert as a team, a youthful level of pregnenolone is absolutely vital.

T3 (triiodothyronine) and **T4** (L-thyroxine) are your basic thyroid hormones. You will get more dramatic effects from raising low thyroid levels than with any other hormone. This is where doctors and endocrinologists are really clueless. Measure your FREE T3 and FREE T4 (and your TSH if you wish). Your free T3 and T4 tell you what you need to know. You want average, midrange values, and not merely "in range" values (add high and low range, and divide by two). Low range values are known as "subclinical hypothyroidism." Doctors rarely measure free T3 and free T4, and they tell you that any in-range value is acceptable. If you are low in either, or both, of these you will get more dramatic results for your money than with any other hormone. *You must treat T3 and T4 separately.* Do not take Armour® or other animal extracts. Use generic versions of Synthroid® and Cytomel®. These are both bioidentical in every way. There is a classic 4:1 ratio in mammals of L-throxine to triiodothyronine. At Lanzhou Medical College the doctors said, "Thyroid hormone levels are closely correlated with age, and age is an independent influencing thyroid hormone factor in patients with essential hypertension." They found T3 and T4 to be very influential here. The same situation was discovered at Harvard University. "The authors have found that free T4 is lower and TSH is higher in hypertensives compared with normo-

67

tensive euthyroid (healthy) subjects." Low thyroid has been associated with aortic stiffness, an important factor in hypertension. Anyone over 40 should know their thyroid hormone levels.

Growth hormone (GH) is very overrated, mostly because it is expensive and some movie stars use it. The only reason it is expensive is because it is very difficult to biosynthesize a 192-amino acid chain molecule. Anyone over 50 can get moderate benefits from using GH. Our levels fall from the time we were teenagers until the time we're 80 or older, when GH almost disappears. Yes, you can get real benefits here if you're willing to pay at least $120 a month for 30 IU. You must inject 1 IU subcutaneously every day. Do not expect anything dramatic here, just because you are spending a lot of money. *Do not even think of taking this until every one of your basic hormones is balanced.* Don't even consider it! It is very difficult to get today unless you pay a doctor and a pharmacist hundreds of dollars a month. Chinese Jintropin® is now off the market, and American doctors use American GH rather than inexpensive Chinese Hypertropin® (formerly Hygertropin).

Estradiol (E2) is the strongest and most dangerous of the three basic estrogens. Men over 50 literally have higher levels of estradiol than their postmenopausal wives! Western women generally have excessive E2 levels due to high fat consumption, obesity, and lack of exercise. These are major causes of breast, cervical, and ovarian cancers. One-third of U.S. women will choose to be castrated, and, then may have low estrogen levels. *All hysterectomies atrophy the ovaries*, which means diminished hormone production. You want low-normal levels here and not just normal ones. At Laiwu People's Hospital (*Fangshe Zazhi* v 19, 2006) both male and female hypertensives were shown to have high estradiol levels. "The authors suggested that the changes of serum sex hormones levels might be a risk factor rather than a consequence of essential hypertension." At the General Hospital in Beijing (*Zhonghua Zazhi* v 9, 2007) men were found to have high estradiol and high estrogen-to-testosterone ratios. Young men have a healthy reversed ratio where testosterone domiates estradiol and estrone; testosterone should dominate.

Estrone (E1) is the second strongest and, potentially, most dangerous of the three basic estrogens. Men over 50 literally have higher levels of estrone than their postmenopausal wives! Supposedly women in America and Europe are estrogen-deficient as they age, and need supplementation of estradiol and estrone. The truth is that Western women generally have excessive E1 levels, due to high fat consumption, obesity, and lack of exercise. This is also a major cause of various female cancers such as uterine, breast, cervical, and ovarian. Since one-third of American women get hysterectomies, many of these women have low estradiol, estrone, estriol, and progesterone levels. Again, you want *low normal levels*, and not just normal ones. What is considered "normal" in Western medicine is actually excessive. Rural Asian and African women have lower estradiol and estrone levels and higher estriol levels. Rural Asian men also have lower estradiol and estrone levels than Westerners.

Estriol, like pregnenolone, is the forgotten or orphan hormone, even though it comprises 80 percent of human estrogen. Doctors almost never test for it, never prescribe it, and the word estriol is really not even in their vocabulary. Studies have shown up to 100 percent of obese women are deficient in estriol. Doctors know nothing about estriol, nor do they care. Amazingly enough you cannot buy or even special order estriol in regular pharmacies! This shows that the pharmaceutical world is in the Dark Ages. Only compounding pharmacies can make this up, but they extort you by selling $1 worth for $50. You can find this on the Internet in 0.3% creams, even though it is not legal to sell it without a prescription. This is the "safe" or "good" estrogen, and Asian and vegetarian women have higher levels. You want high normal levels here and not merely normal ones. You only need about 500 mcg to 1,000 mcg (1 mg) a day in your blood, if you test low by blood or saliva diagnosis.

Cortisol is the stress hormone. Very little work has been done on either lowering or raising cortisol levels. Oral cortisol tablets (Cortef®) are rarely prescribed and hard to find to supplement low cortisol levels. High levels can only be lowered by diet, exercise, and dealing with any stress that is causing them. We need more research on practical application here, since our levels vary widely during a

24-hour period. This is why only a four sample saliva test can give you an accurate profile of this variance. You can do a 12- hour profile at 9/1/5/9, or a 15-hour profile at 8/1/6/11. With most illnesses you do not need to test cortisol, but with hypertension this should be done. Just do a four-sample test over 12 or 15 hours to get an accurate profile. At the 401 Hospital in China (*Zhongguo Kangfu* v 8, 2004) hypertensive men showed high cortisol readings along with depression and anxiety. At the University of New South Wales (*Steroids* v 60, 1995) an extensive review was done with 34 references showing hypertension is highly correlated with high cortisol levels. They said this is characterized by sodium retention. Surprisingly, they did not test the cortisol levels of hypertensive patients. At Hubei Central Hospital (*Fangshe Zazhi* v 20, 2007) patients were tested at 8, 4 and midnight for a daily profile. "Marked elevated plasma cortisol levels were observed in patients with essential hypertension and coronary heart disease." At Kharkov Medical University in Russia (*Problemi Patologil* v 1, 2004) they concluded, "Cortisol may be involved to endocrine control of blood pressure in cooperation with complex of metabolic disorders on hypertension."

Cholesterol is, in fact, the mother hormone from which all the sex hormones are made. This, along with your triglycerides, is the best indicator of coronary heart health. CRP (C-reactive protein) and homocysteine are the other two. Please read my book *Lower Cholesterol Without Drugs* to learn how to maintain low levels using diet, supplements, hormones, exercise, and regular short term fasting. Your total cholesterol level should be about 150 mg/dl. Yes, this is a realistic goal, and billions of rural Asians prove it is. Your triglycerides should be under 100. The ONLY way to raise cholesterol is by eating the saturated animal fat found in red meat, poultry, eggs, and dairy products. Triglycerides are raised by eating too much of any simple sugars including honey or fruit juice.

Total hormone balance is a cornerstone of natural health.

Chapter 14: Home Hormone Testing

You do not need to see a doctor to test most of your hormones. It is very expensive to see one, and they usually have no idea what they're doing regarding natural hormone balance. This includes endocrinologists, naturopaths, holistic physicians, and life extension specialists. Let's go over how to test each of our fourteen hormones.

Insulin is best tested as insulin response. Even if your fasting glucose is 85 or less, you should still get an accurate, non-invasive, inexpensive GTT (glucose tolerance test). Always remember that glucose metabolism and insulin levels are central to maintaining normal blood pressure levels. Insulin resistance and blood sugar dysmetabolism are the basic keys to understanding hypertension. You can get inexpensive, and very accurate, glucose meters at any drug store, but this is just not necessary if you maintain a healthy diet and life style. Ask your doctor for a GTT the next time you have an annual checkup.

Testosterone must be tested for your free, not bound or total form. *You must test only free, unbound, bioavailable testosterone.* Men, for example, should be about 100 on the ZRT saliva scale, and women should be about 20 on the ZRT scale. All saliva and blood results differ; there is no universal standard. Women need a ballpark dose of 150 mcg of testosterone in their blood if they are low. This means a sublingual (or DMSO) dose of 200 mg of enanthate or other common salt, (which contains about 150 mcg of actual testosterone). Men need about 4 mg of enanthate or other common salt sublingually (or in DMSO), which contains about 3 mg of actual testosterone. DMSO solutions are not legal, but you can make them yourself. Transdermal creams and gels generally only deliver about 20% into your blood. This means 80% is wasted. Injections are insanity. Oral testosterone is not absorbed. Nasal sprays are not legal, even by prescription. Compounding pharmacists can provide sublingual drops, or you can make them up yourself. Please read my book *Testosterone Is Your Friend – a Book for Men and Women*.

Androstenedione does not have to be tested by men. Women can test this if they are high or low in either testosterone or DHEA. There is no need to take an androstenedione supplement, even if low, as your testosterone supplement will raise this naturally. Look for the youthful level you had at age 30.

DHEA can be tested with saliva as free DHEA. Look for the youthful level you had at age 30. If low, men can take 25 mg orally, and women half-tablets of 12.5 mg. (Women only have about half men's blood level). It is only about 10 percent absorbed, so men get about 2.5 mg in their blood, and women about 1.25 mg. Men should test about 6 or higher on the ZRT scale, and women about 3. The high teenage levels cannot be regained after the age of 40 as with the other hormones due to metabolic changes as we age.

Melatonin has to be tested at home at 3:00 AM, but the current saliva kits in 2009 are simply not reliable. If you are over 40 men can safely take 3 mg at night only and women can take half tablets of 1.5 mg, as their levels are lower. The media have damned melatonin with faint praise as a mere sleep aid, and for jet lag. The clinical facts are that this is a powerful antioxidant that helps regulate and slow down our biological aging clock. Melatonin has powerful anti-cancer and other dramatic properties. The more we study this, the more impressive the evidence is. Test in darkness or subdued light.

Pregnenolone can be tested by blood, but this is expensive and requires a doctor's visit. The current saliva kits in 2009 are also just not reliable, but better ones for both pregnenolone and melatonin saliva tests should be available anytime. Men over 40 can generally take 50 mg, and women 25 mg. Only about 10 percent will actually be absorbed into your blood. Orally is the only practical way to take pregnenolone (or DHEA), as DMSO and nasal spray are not legal even by prescription, and transdermal does not work well at all since it will not dissolve in vegetable oil, DMSO, or alcohol.

T3 and **T4** cannot currently be tested by saliva. Home blood spot tests cost more than blood draws at a doctor! In 2009 we should again have reliable saliva kits to test for free T3 and T4. Go to Internet sites such as www.healthcheckusa.com to do this inexpensively without a doctor with a real blood draw. You must have mid-range levels, and not merely "in range" levels. You must test your free T3 and free T4 (and TSH if you wish to add that). You can also see a doctor, but clearly demand free T3 and free T4. Again, do not accept "in-range values". There are no universal ranges here, and some labs differ.

GH cannot be tested by saliva, and it may be years before saliva kits are available. Ironically, accurate IGF-1 kits are available. IGF-1 does NOT parallel GH, and anyone who says it does is totally misinformed. You would need to go to a clinic for a 9/1/5/9 four-draw comprehensive profile. None of this is necessary. Are you over 50, and can afford $1,400 a year or more? Then, simply inject (s.c. not i.v.) 1 IU daily. Go by real-world results, rather than blood testing. After using it for 90 days did you lose weight and/or body fat? Did you get stronger as proven by weight lifting? Did your cholesterol and triglycerides fall? It may be possible to use GH sublingually in water or ethanol, but there is no clinical science to verify that. The long 192-amino acid chain molecule will not penetrate the skin, and may not penetrate mucous membranes (nasal or sublingual) very well.

Estradiol (E2) is sometimes needed in women who've had hysterectomies. Use a saliva test kit. *You want low normal values*, not normal or higher. Men do not need to test this, unless they suspect high estrogen levels. If low, use a mere 10 mcg (micrograms) in your blood transdermally, in DMSO, or sublingually. Transdermal patches are very overpriced. *Never use oral estradiol of any type.*

Estrone (E1) is also sometimes needed in women who've had hysterectomies. Use a saliva test kit. *You want low normal values*. Men do not need to test this unless they suspect high estrogen levels. If low, use a mere 100 mcg (micrograms) in your blood transdermally, in DMSO, or sublingually. Transdermal patches are very overpriced. *Never use oral estrone of any type.*

Estriol is very often low in American and European women. Use a saliva test kit. *You want high normal values*. Men do not need to test this. If the test says you are under a certain point, but does not state the actual level, then assume you are low. If low, use 500 to 1,000 mcg (1 mg) transdermally, in DMSO, or sublingually. Patches are not available, and never take oral estriol salts. Estriol is the "safe" or "good" estrogen, but very little research has been done. This is the most abundant estrogen in both men and women. *Never use oral estriol of any type.*

Progesterone does not need to be tested in women over 40, or in men. They just need to use it properly. Any woman who's had a hysterectomy should use this. *Saliva is not the best way to test progesterone*, since it is oil soluble and best measured by (fatty) blood serum, not (watery) blood plasma. Men can use a mere 1/8th-teaspoon five days a week directly on their scrotum. Premenopausal women will use this with their cycle. Remember that most all women over 40 have stopped ovulating and no longer produce any significant amount of progesterone. Many younger women can benefit from using this.

Cortisol, like GH, needs a four draw comprehensive profile. Test this at 9/1/5/9 with a saliva test kit. You will probably get a high level at one time and a low level at another. If you have a high level at one time of the day the only way to lower it is with diet, exercise, life style, and balancing your other hormones. If you are low at one time of the day, consider oral cortisol (hydrocortisone) tablets sold as Cortef®. Cortisol varies greatly in most people during different times of the day. There is little research and little practical application for balancing cortisol. We need a lot more research here for practical means to raise low levels.

Cholesterol can be tested at home fairly accurately with test kits. Doctors can test this along with a comprehensive panel. You can also go to Internet websites like www.healthcheckusa.com to get a comprehensive panel without a doctor. Your level must be about 150 mg/dl, and your triglycerides under 100.

Just remember all your hormones work together as a team, in concert, harmoniously like a symphony orchestra. You need to test and balance all your basic hormones as much as possible, to maintain youthful levels throughout your life.

Chapter 15: Heart and Artery Health Review

This chapter will review what we've just covered in the context of total heart and artery health, and not just the pumping pressures of our blood. A full 83 percent of people over 65 years of age die of some form of heart and artery illness. 68 million Americans have some form of heart disease. Heart attacks, the most common condition, are basically caused by atherosclerosis, or clogged arteries. Stroke is the second most common CHD illness. Only in the last 45 years, since 1965, has the concept of "risk factors" been studied and accepted. In every country on earth the biggest killer of humans by far is coronary heart disease. This is especially true in Russia and the former Russian republics. High consumption of animal foods, saturated fats, calories, simple sugars, refined foods, alcohol, and nicotine are the main factors. Rich countries are always sick countries, despite the elaborate medical care. We have about 1.8 million outright heart attacks every year in the U.S., and almost one-third of those people die. The real point is that most all of this is avoidable.

Blood Pressure is one of the most important risk factors. This entire book has shown how to lower blood pressure naturally. People over 65 sometimes have a condition of high systolic-only blood pressure with a systolic reading of 160 or higher, but a near normal diastolic of 90 or less. You must keep your pressures at 120/80 or lower.

Total Cholesterol (TC) should be about 150. Yes, that is a practical level if you're not eating meat, poultry, eggs, or dairy. *TC is the single most important indicator of CHD health.* Rural Asians in general have these low levels. American adults, on average, have high levels of about 240. People who tell you, "cholesterol doesn't count" are obviously wrong. Look at the chart below from the MRFIT Study to prove this beyond any doubt. This involved over a third of a million real men, and cannot be disputed. You want high levels of high density cholesterol (HDL) and low levels of low density (LDL) cholesterol. You really do not need to be overly concerned with your HDL and LDL, as only diet and life style are going to optimize them.

Some self appointed "experts" even tell you that low cholesterol is bad for you. Billions of Asians prove quite the opposite. *The ideal is 150*, and science has proven this repeatedly. Some elderly, sickly people are unable to make much cholesterol despite their high fat diets. In such cases low levels are meaningless. CHD rates fall 2% for every 1% drop in TC. That is very impressive.

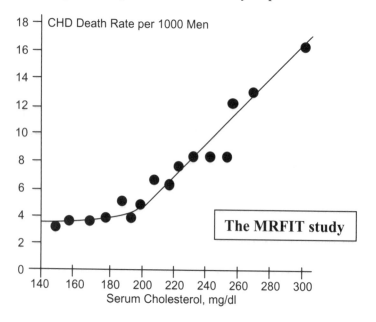

Triglycerides are a secondary, but very important indicator of CHD health, and should be under 100. Here, simple sugars of any kind are the cause of high triglycerides. Americans commonly have levels of 150, due in large part to their intake of 160 pounds each year of sugar in some form. Fat and sugar work synergistically in our bodies to raise triglyerides. This is why vegetarians often have high triglycerides, but low cholesterol; most all of them are sugar addicts.

Homocysteine is a very accurate and proven marker of CHD health in general. This should be under 10 mmol, and preferably well under 10. **C-reactive protein** (high-sensitivity CRP) is a time-proven inflammation marker for heart and artery health. You must keep this under 3 mg/dl on a 1.0-3.0 scale. **Uric acid** is only elevated by eating animal protein from meat, poultry, eggs, and dairy. Your level should be under 5 mg/dl. Get these three tests done during your annual physical.

Blood sugar, insulin, and insulin resistance are very powerful influences on CHD. Your fasting blood sugar must be 85 or less. **85 is the Magic Number**, not the usual figure of 100 that the doctor will tell you. Again, it is more accurate to get an inexpensive GTT test rather than test insulin levels per se. Do not accept a GTT level over 100, as the usual accepted level of 110 just isn't low enough.

Anyone over the age of 50, or who suspects any heart problem at all, should seriously consider an inexpensive, non-invasive electro-cardiogram (EKG/ECG). This should be standard procedure for this age group. It will reveal hidden and unsuspected problems, especially left ventricular hypertrophy, and is well worth doing. Age itself is one of the most important factors. The older you are the more heart and artery disease you'll have. Race and genetics are other unchangeable factors. White Europeans are the most prone to heart disease. It is well-known that you are more prone if either of your parents had heart disease. Age, genetics, and race are givens.

Trans-fats (aka hydrogenated fats), deserve special mention. You must avoid all hydrogenated fats and oils. These are synthetic chemical creations that clog your arteries. Science has proven that they should never be fed to humans or animals. The University of Kuopio in Finland fed people a mere 5 percent hydrogenated oil in their food for only a month. They found serious negative effects, especially with cholesterol and triglycerides. Tufts University in Boston, Wegeningen University in the Netherlands, and the University of Oslo are among the hundreds of clinics internationally that have verified this. Harvard Medical School said, *"Hydrogenated fats are directly related to risk of CHD."* Consumption of these has also been clearly connected to various cancer rates. Margarine is far worse than butter. Read your labels, and never buy or eat anything that contains these chemical abominations. Read your labels.

Proven supplements are very important, but secondary to diet. The supplements were discussed in Chapter 8: Proven Supplements. If you are over 40, take most all of these for total holistic health. *Treat your whole body, and not just your cardiovascular system.* The most important heart healthy supplements are beta-sitosterol, vitamins, minerals, flax oil, vitamin D, soy isoflavones, and carnosine.

Hormones are far more important to heart health than the medical profession realizes. Our endocrine system strongly influences our heart and artery functions. These are discussed in Chapter 13: Your Basic Hormones. The medical profession still holds onto the irrational myth that testosterone is heart unhealthy, while estrogen is heart healthy. Quite the opposite is true, as we've shown. Men do have more heart disease, and women do live six years longer than men on average. It will continually be emphasized that all our hormones work together in harmony, synergistically together as a team. We have fourteen basic hormones that should be balanced, especially after the age of 40. We know youthful levels of T3, T4, testosterone, and DHEA support good CHD health. High levels of estradiol and estrone, on the other hand, are unhealthy. Our other hormones may not have as much direct influence, but *it is just as important to balance them as part of the whole hormone team.* Science will soon prove their value in heart and artery health, too.

Exercise has to be emphasized. We all know exercise is heart healthy, but most people don't get nearly enough of it. Most Westerners do not do physical labor anymore, but rather more sedentary, technical jobs. You can do resistance or aerobic, and ideally both of these. Over 30 years ago Nathan Pritikin put very sickly heart patients on a low fat, near-macrobiotic diet based on whole grains. He had them walk as much as they safely could. He got miracles from this simple two step regimen! If he were alive today, and had the hormones and supplements we have now, he would get even faster and more dramatic miracles. Walking is the best and most practical exercise of all.

Obesity is very closely related to heart and artery diseases rates. There is abdominal ("male") obesity, and hips/buttocks ("female") obesity. Americans eat twice the calories they need, eight times the fat they need (42%), the worst kinds of fats, 160 pounds of various sugars we don't need at all, refined foods, chemicalized, and preserved foods. It's not just that obesity causes higher rates of CHD, but that it causes skyrocketing medical costs, poor quality of life, and much earlier death. *Obesity is a major cause of all-cause mortality.* Obesity is correlated with every known medical condition and illness (except osteoporosis). This is agreed on by the international scientists. One typical example is Tohuku University in Japan where studies found statistically significant relationships between excess body weight and increased medical costs, all-cause mortality, and risk of cancer incidence.

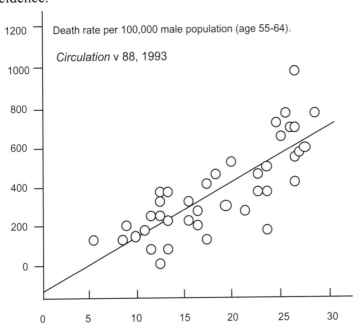

Cholesterol Saturated Fat Index per 1000 kcal/day
The more saturated fat you eat the more coronary
heart disease you get based on 40 countries.

Look at the chart above to prove that the more animal fat you eat the more heart disease you get. Diet and life style, together, is the only way to keep your heart strong and your arteries clear. This was discussed in Chapter 5: Diet, Diet, Diet. Your worst enemy here, is animal fat and animal protein. *Fat intake must be limited to 10% to*

20%, and no more. This should all be vegetable oils ideally, and not animal fats. Use such oils as sunflower, safflower, corn, and olive, in moderation. Avoid canola oil (there are no canola plants!), as it is another chemical aberration full of toxic erucic acid. If you insist on eating meat, poultry, or eggs you must limit these to 10 percent of your diet, or one four-ounce serving a day. Dairy should be omitted completely, even the low-fat and no-fat varieties.

Fasting is the most powerful healing method known to man. Fasting one day a week, from dinner to dinner on a given day, is very effective in that you get fifty-two short fasts every year. You can also join our monthly Young Again two-day fast, on the last weekend of every month. Fasting will strengthen your heart and help clear your arteries.

Diabetes has more bad effect than any other illness. The American Diabetes Association defines this as a blood sugar level of 126 mg/dl or higher. One in three American children will grow up diabetic. This is hard to even comprehend.

Smoking is a very powerful contributor to CHD deaths. Male smokers have ten times the basic heart disease rate, and women five times. It is estimated that one third of the heart attacks every year are largely due to smoking. Drinking alcohol in excess of two drinks a day has a negative effect, but none if less than that. However, even two drinks a day causes other health problems. Coffee does not have a strong effect on CHD, but there are many other reasons not to drink it, or to at least limit it to one cup a day.

It should be emphasized that lowering any of these factors with prescription drug therapy does not reduce CHD rates at all. Those must be improved with diet and life style. Taking statin drugs does not lengthen life, but does make your overall health worse. The side effects are very serious. Taking antihypertensive drugs will superficially lower your blood pressure, but not add to the years you live. Americans take more prescription drugs than any other country.

80

Chapter 16: Bad Habits

One of the *Seven Steps to Natural Health* (listed on page 85) is to limit or stop any bad habits. One doesn't have to be a saint, but you do have to be sincere. You don't have to live the life of an ascetic, but you just can't blindly indulge in whatever you like to do. Freedom is not doing what you want, but *doing what is best*. Will power is an illusion, and no amount of imagined "will power" is going to stop you from bad habits. *Insight is the key*. Understanding brings freedom from bad habits. When you actually realize how harmful sugar, alcohol, nicotine, caffeine, and most recreational drugs are, you will stop using or abusing them. Bad habits just encourage more bad habits.

The main bad habit is sugar addiction. Americans gulp down over 160 pounds of various simple sugars every year. This is an addiction, plain and simple. This insane intake of sugar causes high blood sugar and insulin resistance. Insulin resistance is the key to understanding hypertension, and simple carbohydrates (sugars) are the basic cause of blood sugar disorders of all types. Ten per cent fresh (or frozen) fruit is all you can safely eat, and many people should just stop eating fruit altogether. Fruit simply just has no real nutrition to speak of, and is basically sugar, water, and a little fiber. There are almost no minerals or vitamins in any fruit. Read the article *Fruits Have Almost No Nutrition* at my website <u>www.youngagain.org</u>.

The four other bad habits come down to alcohol, nicotine, caffeine, and various prescription and recreational drugs. Yes, taking prescription drugs is a bad habit, too. There is a huge volume of literature on the first three, but very little on prescription drugs, marijuana, cocaine, ecstasy, amphetamines, opiates, or the psychedelic drugs. One of the *Seven Steps to Natural Health* is no prescription drugs; this includes recreational ones as well.

Let's start with alcohol. The most popular and destructive drug in the entire world. People of European descent are the most resistant to alcohol damage, while Asian, Blacks, American Indians, and others are far more susceptible to the effects. *The more alcohol you drink the higher you can expect your blood pressure to go.* Alcoholics have inordinately high rates. When they stop drinking, their pressures immediately drop significantly, and stay lower. Studies in the *Lancet* (v 1, 1984), *Hypertension* (v 44, 2004 and v 9, 1987), and the book *Hypertension* (Klatsky 2000) all show very clearly that there is a direct correlation between how many drinks you have and how high your pressures are. You can get by with one daily drink, but not by going seven days without any and then having those seven drinks on the weekend. Let's be clear, alcohol is a biological poison, and some people should never drink at all.

There is no "French Paradox!" Alcohol is proven to cause liver damage, and many other problems. Some studies have even claimed that eliminating alcohol is more important than exercising. On the other hand, a few other studies have shown that people who drink 1 or 2 drinks a day had equal or even lower pressures than non-drinkers. At Kyushi University it was found that even light drinking raised blood pressure in Japanese people. At Yamagata University, alcohol response was shown to be a largely genetic factor. Epidemiological studies over the last quarter-century prove beyond any doubt the relationship of alcohol intake and hypertension, especially heavier drinking. Blood pressure falls within days after the cessation of alcohol, and rises within days when it is resumed. Some people can drink in moderation (e.g. one drink a day), while others are simply too alcohol sensitive, and too predisposed to alcoholism. Just three or more drinks daily for men and two or more drinks for women is considered "heavy" drinking. Drinking also contributes to obesity, and obesity is another very basic factor here. All these are well established, inarguable facts.

A study in the *American Journal of Clinical Nutrition* (v 87, 2008) found alcohol contributed to Metabolic Syndrome or pre-diabetes. The more people drank, the more prone to diabetes and insulin resistance they were. At the University of Barcelona (*Hypertension* v 33, 1999) men who drank over 100 g (about 3.3 oz) of pure ethanol daily (one cup of 80 proof liquor) were admitted to their clinic, where they stopped drinking. In one month their systolic pressure fell an average of 7.2 mm, and their diastolic 6.6 mm. Their heart rate also decreased significantly. On admission, 42 percent were diagnosed with clinical hypertension, but after only 30 days this fell to 12 percent. This is amazing. It was done with no change in diet or exercise, but just the elimination of all alcohol. The University of Texas verified these findings (*Hypertension* v 39, 2002).

It seems the entire world is addicted to the caffeine in coffee and tea, and this may be the most popular drug of all. The explosion of energy drinks in the last few years has greatly expanded the use of caffeine, especially among younger people who don't drink coffee. At Okayama University the researchers found that caffeine is an angiotensin blocker and increases blood pressure 5 to 10 mmHg. This is very clear. At the University of Oklahoma the doctors warned that caffeine is an important contributor to the extreme incidence of hypertension in our country, and should be curtailed. Caffeine raises blood pressure by elevating vascular resistance. The pressor response to caffeine occurs equally in persons at rest and under stress. Again, at this university caffeine was given to five distinct hypertension groups. Caffeine raised both systolic and diastolic blood pressure in all groups. The largest study of all, from the University of Helsinki, studied 24,710 healthy Finnish people, not on hypertensive drugs or with any known CHD conditions. The results indicated that coffee drinking increases the risk of hypertensive drug treatment, and this risk was higher in subjects with low-to-moderate coffee intakes. We get the same results from the Israeli Hypertension Institute, Duke University, and other clinics around the world. The most comprehensive study came from the University of Utrect. Coffee abstinence was associated with a lower hypertension risk than was low coffee consumption. Even a little regular coffee has strong negative effects.

There is very little information about the use of tobacco and nicotine on blood pressure. Some studies found it raised pressure, while other studies actually found a lowering effect. The doctors at Dongguk University in South Korea claimed cigarette smoking acutely increases arterial stiffness and blood pressure in male smokers with hypertension, and the effects persist longer than in male smokers without hypertension. The San Diego campus of the University of California showed that smoking clearly raises homocysteine levels

(9.5 vs 7.9 mmol). Oestra Hospital in Sweden claimed that smokers had significantly lower systolic (but not diastolic) blood pressures. The Centre de Recherche Clinique said that even former smokers have definitely higher rates of hypertension than never smokers.

Americans take far more prescription drugs than anyone else. The most popular are anti-depressants (Xanax, Valium, and others) and opiates (codeine, hydrocodone, oxycodone, and morphine). *Hydrocodone* (such as Vicodin®) *is the most prescribed drug in America*, with over 100 million prescriptions a year. That's right, hydrocodone* is the most prescribed drug in America. Opiates are not toxic if used in moderation, because they are plant based. Such drugs as Valium just seem to be perennial favorites. The misuse of prescription drugs is epidemic in America. There is just no reason to take prescription drugs, except temporarily in emergencies (and rare cases such as insulin for type 1 diabetics). The regular use of toxic, synthetic, chemical poisons will only make your health problems worse.

Recreational, non-prescription drug use is also an epidemic. Marijuana is all too popular among people of all ages. Fortunately, this causes little physical harm if used moderately. The problem is that it causes psychological and mental deterioration, including apathy, lack of motivation, forgetfulness, and mental fogginess. Ecstasy is a modified amphetamine, and is very toxic. Amphetamine and methamphetamine users often become dependent or addicted, and ruin their bodies, their minds, and their very lives. Cocaine is as addictive as it is overrated - *the drug of illusion*. In countries like Peru, where it is legal, people drink coca tea. They are as dependent as people are dependent on coffee, but there is no antisocial or criminal activity associated with it. Cocaine use has been strongly associated with hypertension and heart disease in general. Psychedelics largely went out of favor after the early 1970s. There is almost no biological damage here, but the mental effects from them are powerful, mostly due to insincere use. Dependence on anything harms you.

In America all forms of hydrocodone contain large amounts of toxic acetominophen or aspirin, which cause far, far more damage than the drug itself.

Seven Steps to Natural Health

With these seven steps you can cure "incurable" illnesses like cancer, diabetes, heart disease, and others naturally without drugs, surgery, or chemotherapy. These are seven vital steps to take if you want optimum health and long life. Do your best to do all of them. The only step to add would be prayer or meditation.

- An American macrobiotic whole grain based diet is central to everything. Diet cures disease; everything else is secondary.

- Proven supplements are powerful when you're eating right. There are only about twenty scientifically proven supplements for those over forty, and eight for those under forty.

- Natural hormone balance is the third step. The fourteen basic hormones are listed on page 62. You can do this inexpensively without a doctor.

- Exercise is vital, even if it is just a half-hour of walking a day. Whether it is aerobic or resistance you need to exercise regularly.

- Fasting is the most powerful healing method known to man. Just fast from dinner to dinner on water one day a week. Join our monthly Young Again two day fast. The fasting calendar is at www.youngagain.org the last weekend of every month.

- No prescription drugs, except *temporary* antibiotics or pain medication during an emergency. (There are rare exceptions such as insulin for type 1 diabetics who have no operant pancreas.)

- The last step is to limit or end any bad habits such as alcohol, coffee, recreational drugs, or desserts. You don't have to be a saint, but you do need to be sincere.

85

Other Books by Safe Goods

The Natural Prostate Cure – Roger Mason	$ 6.95 US
The Minerals You Need – Roger Mason	$ 4.95 US
What is Beta Glucan? – Roger Mason	$ 4.95 US
Lower Cholesterol without Drugs – Roger Mason	$ 6.95 US
The Natural Diabetes Cure – Roger Mason	$ 8.95 US
No More Horse Estrogen! – Roger Mason	$ 7.95 US
Zen Macrobiotics for Americans – Roger Mason	$ 7.95 US
Testosterone Is Your Friend- Roger Mason	$ 8.95 US
The ADD and ADHD Diet Expanded	$10.95 US
ADD, The Natural Approach	$ 5.95 US
Eye Care Naturally	$ 8.95 US
The Smart Brain Train	$ 7.95 US
New Hope for Serious Diseases	$ 7.95 US
Cancer Disarmed Expanded	$ 7.95 US
The Vertical System	$ 9.95 US
Overcoming Senior Moments Expanded	$ 9.95 US
The Secrets of Staying Young	$11.95 US
Worse Than Global Warming	$ 9.95 US
2012 Airborne Prophesy	$16.95 US
Rx for Computer Eyes	$ 8.95 US
Kids First: Health with No Interference	$16.95 US
Prevent Cancer, Strokes, Heart Attacks	$11.95 US

For a complete listing of books visit our web site:
www.safegoodspub.com to order, or call (888) 628-8731/
(888) NATURE-1 for a free catalog